SONG OF THE SPINE

by
June Leslie Wieder

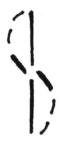

Published and distributed by

Booksurge Publishing LLC
5341 Dorchester Road
Suite 16
North Charleston, SC 29418
866-308-6235
www.booksurge.com

Books may be ordered via the Internet from
www.bone-toning.com or www.drwieder.com

Song of the Spine
Copyright © 2004 by June Leslie Wieder

All rights reserved. No part of this book may be copied or reproduced in any form or by any means or stored in an electronic system without permission in writing from the author (contact via e-mail: doctajune@aol.com).

This book is an informational guide to bone toning and vibrational medicine. Techniques and approaches described in this book should not be used to treat physical or medical problems without prior consultation with a qualified healthcare professional.

Images from the book *Cymatics: A Study of Wave Phenomena and Vibration* (© 2001, Macromedia Publishing), by Hans Jenny, are used by permission.

ISBN 1-59457-470-7

Printed in the United States of America

CONTENTS

	Preface	v
1	Song of the Spine	1
2	Harmonic Healing – A Brief History	7
3	The Soul of Harmony and the Science of Harmonics	21
4	Some Modern Sound Therapies	37
5	Sound Creates Form	49
6	Bone Toning	59
7	Muscle Testing	75
8	Procedures, Case Histories, and Research	85
9	Vibration in Conventional Medicine	93
10	Neurobiology of Vibrational Healing	101
11	Future Directions	119
12	The Dance of Life	123
	Suggested Readings and Other Sources	125
	Recommended Websites	129

PREFACE

THIS BOOK IS THE RESULT of many years of research, experiencing, and experimenting with sound-health. I began chanting when I was a child, and today chanting is an integral part of my life.

While working in a psychiatric ward, I came to realize the valuable role that music and sound play in our day-to-day health and our well-being. When I played the piano for and with patients, we shared a universal language. The emotions we felt were penetrating and expressed enthusiastically.

This book represents a small fraction of the grandeur that is to be found in our harmonious nature, which pervades everything. I sincerely hope that this book helps to illuminate and stimulate the minds of seekers of truth, and that it will open your heart to the realization that we are all one, yet we each pulse to our own beat.

It is my deepest belief that every cell in our bodies represents a point of light in the heavens that sings its song of praise to life.

Breathe deeply. Enjoy the journey!

*　*　*

I gratefully acknowledge all those pioneers who were courageous enough to put forth their ideas about vibrational healing, all the musicians who have given us the experience of expanded consciousness, all the scientists and researchers who have given us greater insight in the field of vibrational medicine, and all the teachers and writers who devoted their lives to sharing this knowledge.

My heartfelt gratitude goes to my family, mentors, and friends – Carol and William Wieder, Yaacov Wieder, the late Milton Trager, M.D., Gail Stewart, Dr. David Donaldson, Dr. Charles "Skip" Lantz, Jonathan and Andi Goldman, Sarah Benson, Joshua Leeds, and Shirley Helmick.

Special thanks to my copy editor, Jill Breedon, for her careful work in preparing my manuscript for publication, and to my consulting editors, Matthew Jon Prest and Richard P. Leavitt; and most heartfelt thanks to my chief editor, dear friend, and heartpartner, David Pope, for without Dezrt Dave this book would not have been possible.

For artwork I thank Suzi O'Grady and for the cover art Marcia Didtler. I would also like to thank Major Tom for digitizing the cover illustration, and N. Kay Farrell of Graphic Impressions and Steve Davis, life coach and trainer at FacilitatorU.com, for the final cover design.

Loving thanks to those friends who have given tone, rhythm, and harmony to my life: Dr. Matthew Jon Prest, Patrick Michael Escott, Andrew Mitchell, Frank Rowicki, Sean Gallagher, Miron Mercury, Glenn Matson, Herm Peterson, Dr. Steve Angel, Louise Knecht, Louise Kelar, Julie Robinson, Ruthie Mae Lichten, and Teresa Holzer.

Deepest thanks to all my patients who moved me to seek finer sound solutions.

CHAPTER 1

SONG OF THE SPINE

In the beginning
there was the word
the sound
the Song

IN ALL CREATION, animals communicate with sounds and songs. The humpback sings beautiful songs that sound very much like human ballads. It is only male humpback whales that are known to sing, and their songs are like a deep, haunting mournful raga that once heard cannot be forgotten. These songs contain complex vibrational patterns, and although the humpback is capable of singing over a range of seven octaves (similar to the range of the piano), it typically sings notes belonging to only one octave. Like humans, whales use rhythm to remember their songs from season to season. Scientists believe that humpbacks use their songs to communicate with one another over hundreds or even thousands of miles. In some Native American cultures, it is said that whale medicine shamans have the ability to tap into universal consciousness.

Other mammals, such as bats, emit a steady stream of high-frequency ultrasonic clicks or chirps, up to 200,000 times per second. Electronic devices are needed to reduce these ultrasonic sounds to frequencies our ears can hear. Bats use echolocation to find their way and their prey. These echolocation chirps are like musical notes, so that the bat receives a "musical" picture.

The timing of the echoes composes an image of the landscape that describes the type of prey, the direction of its movement, and its velocity. Medical researchers are now developing a navigation device for blind persons that emits ultrasonic bat-like calls and converts the echoes into sounds that can be heard by the person using the device. Preliminary tests of the device show that humans adapt remarkably well to the bat echo-location system.

The American Museum of Natural History once had an alligator named Oscar that would bellow a B-flat whenever it heard a B-flat played on any kind of instrument. Some observers believe that the B-flat bellow is used by alligators as a mating call. But perhaps the alligator's B-flat bellow is something much more primordial. Astronomers have recently discovered that a black hole in the Perseus star cluster emits a B-flat sound wave 57 octaves below the middle B-flat on a piano.

Birds compose songs using various rhythms, changing pitches and permutations. Citing the work of the late Luis Baptista, Patricia Gray (head of the biomusic program at the National Academy of the Sciences) wrote, "The canyon wren's trill cascades down the musical scale like the opening of Chopin's *Revolutionary Etude*." Baptista's analysis revealed that the canyon wren sings in a chromatic scale, which divides the octave into 12 semitones. Birds can identify a wide range of frequencies and remember their arrangement. Within a bird's song, many frequencies or tones may be sounded simultaneously, and quite different birdcalls may sound the same to our ears. A bird's brain can distinguish between the subtle rise and fall of pitches, perceive the changes in the sound's shape, and listen for repetitive patterns. So the next time you are called a birdbrain, take it as a compliment!

An ancient Chinese proverb says: "A bird does not sing because it has an answer – it sings because it has a song."

Is it coincidental that many different species share a similar pattern of songs and melodies? I think not.

Music calls to the heart of our emotions. Music can bring tears of joy or tears of sadness. The appreciation of music is universal and profound. The question remains whether there is any evolutionary advantage to the songs of humans and other animals. In searching for answers, many scientists are delving into the origins and purpose of music.

Could it be that music predates human civilization or language? I think so. Flutes made by Neanderthals more than 43,000 years ago have been recovered in France and Slovenia by paleoanthropologists.

Where in the brain is music processed? Are there specialized neurons that interpret music? According to Daniel J. Levitin and other researchers, when a person listens to music, neural structures in the cerebellar vermis, a primitive region of the brain, are activated. Because music so profoundly affects our emotions, Levitin suspects that it must have some ancient and important function.

Levitin proposes that music stimulates our innate drive to find patterns in the environment. He writes, "From our culture we learn (even if unconsciously) about musical structures, tones, and other ways of understanding music as it unfolds over time, and brains are exercised by extracting different patterns." He also suggests that music may serve as a means of communication.

The father of chiropractic, Daniel David Palmer, stated that "Chiropractic is founded on tone." When the spine loses its "tone," the result can be what chiropractors call a subluxation, a partial dislocation of the vertebrae that affects the nervous system and surrounding tissues. There are 12 vertebrae in the primary or kyphotic (thoracic) curve, which starts at the T1 vertebra and runs through to T12. The secondary or lordotic (neck and lower back) curves also have a total of 12 vertebrae.

It dawned on me that the spine, with its kyphotic and lordotic curves, looks like a standing wave. A standing or stationary wave consists of a wave and its reflection. Energy is transferred back and forth between the two parts of the wave. Is it possible, I thought, that some kind of energy echoes between the primary and secondary curves of the spine in order to maintain the structural and neural integrity of the spine and nervous system?

That question led to a long period of research into the resonance of the spine. From physics, I learned that any object that vibrates has its own natural resonance and that the range of the resonance can be broad or narrow. When an object encounters vibrations that are within its natural frequency, it will begin to oscillate and produce vibrations that augment the original vibrations. I thought that a vertebra, like most objects, is likely to have a natural resonance. Because the vertebrae of the spine differ in size, shape, and weight, each vertebra is likely to have its own natural frequency of vibration.

My first step was to determine the resonant frequency of each vertebra. Because of my background in music, I quite naturally thought of using tuning forks to apply different frequencies to the vertebrae. I used a technique called muscle testing to determine if a specific frequency had a strong effect when applied to a vertebra. Muscle testing is a comprehensive yet exquisitely specific system for discovering the innate resonance of the whole person.

I used 12 tuning forks, one for each of the 12 semitones in the octave. I applied each of the 12 tuning forks individually to each of the 24 vertebrae, and performed muscle testing during each application. The results were remarkable: for each vertebra, only one of the tuning forks resulted in a strong muscle-test response, and the remaining 11 tuning forks produced weak responses.
In other words, each bone of the spine has its own tone and frequency. These tones of the 24 movable vertebrae form what I call the *Song of the Spine*.

The next step was to determine if applying specific vibrational frequencies to the vertebrae would generate a sympathetic response that would activate these embedded harmonics that lie within the spine. In many cases, the results have been astounding. I call this vibrational therapy *bone toning*. It is my great hope that this book will stimulate and encourage others to experience the power of sound healing, and further investigate the therapeutic uses of sound.

Although tuning forks have proved to be an effective tool for restoring harmonic resonance in the spine, using them for extended periods of time is not very practical. So I commissioned an electronics engineer to build a device that generates the specific vibrational frequency that I found corresponding to the bones of the spine – a device that can easily be applied to any location on the spine. Such a frequency generator will soon be available to researchers and practitioners.

Every system in the body has a rhythmical nature and inherent harmony. This rhythmic harmony is expressed, for example, in the expansion and contraction of the diaphragm, the beating of the heart, and the circulation of the cerebrospinal fluid from the skull to the sacrum. And to all this, we can now add the *Song of the Spine*.

CHAPTER 2

HARMONIC HEALING – A BRIEF HISTORY

**Each illness is a musical problem – the healing,
a musical solution. The shorter and more complete
the solution – the greater the musical talent of
the physician. Sickness demands manifold solutions.
The selection of the most appropriate solution determines
the talent of the physician.**
   —*From Novalis, an 18th-century German mystic poet*

IN ANCIENT GREECE, Apollo was the god of music, medicine, and poetry. He was the Olympian god of Harmony. According to Greek legend, Apollo created the cithara (pronounced kithara), a stringed instrument on which the modern guitar is based. Apollo, it is said, also gave Orpheus the lyre, a harp-like stringed instrument, and the Muses taught Orpheus how to play it. There were nine Muses, each of whom presided over a different art or science. Orpheus eventually gained the power to play music so sweet that it could sway men and gods, enchant plants, and even stir inanimate objects. The Greek term *Muses* is the origin of the English word *music*.

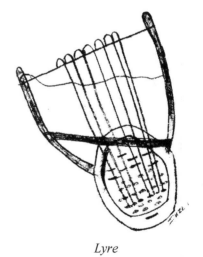

Lyre

Pythagoras (582–507 BC), the renowned Greek mathematician, musician, mystic, teacher, philosopher, and prophet, thought that the universe embodied numerical symmetries with perfect geometric proportions that could be expressed as ratios. He used the Greek word *kosmos*, which implies harmony and order, to describe what we today call the universe. Pythagoras, although he is best known to us for his mathematics, actually founded a school to study musical harmony and geometry. He believed that the perfect and harmonious proportions of the *kosmos* could be re-created in music, particularly the divine sounds created by the planetary spheres, which in later centuries came to be known as the "Music of the Spheres."

Before Pythagoras, Sumerian and Taoist doctrines dating back more than 6,000 years refer to the idea that harmony exists everywhere, including the heavens. In ancient Egypt, a precursor to Pythagoras – Hermes Trismegistus – was known both as the Egyptian god Thoth and in human form as a prophet, in the time of Pharaoh Ammon. The writings of Hermes were consulted by Pythagoras. One of the famous Hermetic principles states, "As above, so below." The surviving Hermetic texts include descriptions of how to use music to carry cosmic energy and tones down to Earth.

To the Pythagoreans, Apollo symbolized a harmonic nature that could be expressed through music. Pythagoras felt that music used in the right way could contribute greatly to a person's health. Some consider him to be the originator of musical medicine. The Pythagoreans were perhaps the first musical theorists, and they developed a numerical method for describing musical intervals. At that time, the cithara was used for musical accompaniment, and it is thought that the players of the cithara used a scale that is very similar to our modern musical scale.

Like the Greeks, the ancient cultures of Judaism, Buddhism, and Hinduism held that music is an expression of natural harmonics. They all recognized that music consists of complex relationships that connect many elements. All of these cultures used music and sounds as a method of healing.

The music of the Jewish people is like a rich and colorful tapestry that illustrates their historical struggles. Their melodies carry with them the depth of their oppression and the celebration of their freedom. Music has played an important role in the history of the Jewish people for more than 2,500 years. There are many references to music in the Torah; for example, when the Children of Israel made their exodus from Egypt, they sang in celebration of their escape as Miriam danced on the shores of the Red Sea.

God's last commandment to Moses for the Jewish people was to copy the Torah, which God called a song: "Now write for yourselves this Song and teach it" (Deuteronomy 31:19). An enlightened rabbi named Akiva said this of the Torah: "Sing it every day, sing it every day." Music is referred to more often in the historical texts of the Jewish people than in those of almost any other culture.

Sound has been used as a transformational agent by aboriginal cultures in Africa, Asia, America, and the Pacific. From prehistoric times until today, tribes have used chanting, drumming, and a variety of musical instruments to uplift the spirit and to promote healing. In healing ceremonies throughout the world, medicine men, or shamans, have used and still use sound to heal. Shamans often regard illness as being caused by imbalance or disharmony in the body or spirit, and they typically use drums, rattles, or other musical accompaniment to restore the natural harmony of the body.

With the aid of chanting and dancing, the shaman tries to contact guardian spirits who can help to heal the individual. The word "shaman" is of Siberian origin. In some parts of the world, a shaman is regarded as a sorcerer or a seer. Such shamans have developed methods for creating visions in which they visit the spirit realm. The shaman shifts into different states of consciousness and travels to other realms to contact guardian spirits that can aid in the healing of others. To invoke these helpful spirits, shamans usually chant.

Chanting is vocalizing in a repetitive fashion, using the principle of harmonics, usually to invoke God or deities. The power of chanting lies in the intention conveyed within these sounds.

The rattle is one of the oldest instruments and has been used for ceremonial and healing work throughout the world. Its purpose is to awaken spiritual energy, disperse negative energies, and connect the consciousness of the individual to the cosmos.

In East Asia, gongs are believed to resonate harmonically with the vibrational frequencies of the cosmos. Gongs have such richness and depth of sound that they are thought to be capable of tuning and aligning the body on a cellular level.

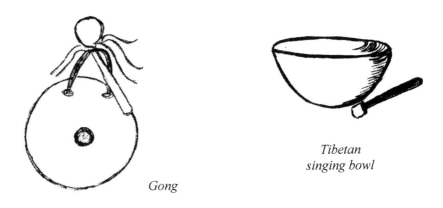

Gong

Tibetan singing bowl

Tibetan singing bowls are made up of seven different metals that correspond to the seven inner planets of our solar system. Like gongs, Tibetan singing bowls are used to realign and balance the physical and energetic fields of the body.

In the Hindu religion, the god Vishnu is depicted as blowing into conch shells to defeat and dispel demons.

Chimes are often used to lighten dense energy patterns and to repair damage to the body's energy fields. Often, chimes are used by practitioners to denote the beginning and the end of a healing session.

Among Australian aboriginals, an instrument called the didgeridoo is used in healing ceremonies. It is thought to ground the physical body. The deep, haunting sound of the didgeridoo opens the gateway to dreamtime, an altered state of consciousness.

Drums represent the beat of the heart, the beat of the Earth. Not surprisingly, they have been used by many ancient cultures in their healing ceremonies. Drums are seen as a means of grounding the body's energy. Even today, the drum is used to synchronize and entrain our breath and heartbeat.

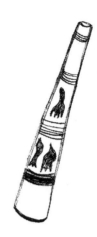

Didgeridoo

Research conducted in the 1970s found that the beating of a drum releases endorphins within us and aids in harmonizing neural activity. At a U.S. Senate hearing on the elderly, Mickey Hart, the drummer for the Grateful Dead and author of the book *Drumming on the Edge of Magic*, described how drumming can been used among older people to promote healing, because drumming is easy enough for almost anyone to do.

"Our bodies," said Hart, "are multidimensional rhythm machines with everything pulsing in synchrony, from the digesting activity of our intestines to the firing of neurons in the brain. Within the body, the main beat is laid down by the cardiovascular system, the heart and the lungs. As we age, however, these rhythms can fall out of sync. And then, suddenly, there is no more important or crucial issue than regaining that lost rhythm."

Power of Chanting

Traditionally throughout the world, chanting has been used to restore inner harmony. The controlled use of the breath in chanting has many beneficial physiological effects, such as slowing down the heart rate, decreasing blood pressure, and improving lung function. Chanting is very simple to learn and can be a powerful tool for entering into a more harmonic state. The repetition of a phrase or a syllable often allows one to invoke a deity, with the intention of becoming one with the source and its creation. The prayers of both Muslims and Jews employ a combined form of chanting and toning. Virtually every religious or spiritual group sings praises using mantras or chants.

Buddhists have developed chanting into a high art. Today, many people in America and Europe have adopted the Buddhist *om* chant. Some prefer to give the word the more phonetic spelling of *aum*: The *a* is pronounced *ah* – the beginning of the breath; the *u* is pronounced with a prolonged sound, with full breath extension, until the final letter *m* is sounded as a humming vibration representing the last stage of the breath. Thus, when we chant *om* or *aum*, it becomes the natural sound of our breath. In Hinduism, *aum* represents the three aspects of God – Brahma, Vishnu, and Shiva.

The Roman Catholic Church has a long tradition of chanting. Perhaps most well-known are the Gregorian chants, so called because Pope Gregory I collected them from many cultures about 600 AD. It is said that Gregorian monks experience the essence of God while they are chanting.

The power of chanting was inadvertently revealed at a Benedictine monastery in France in the 1960s. A young new abbot wanted to modernize the procedures in the monastery and decided to eliminate the daily Gregorian chants, which took up to eight hours a day and left the monks with only a few hours for sleep. Within a short time after the chanting had been terminated, the monks began exhibiting severe fatigue and depression, and became unable to carry out their normal duties. The increased hours of sleep only seemed to exacerbate their fatigue. The abbot called in medical specialists, but none were able to help until Alfred Tomatis – an otolaryngologist and originator of the Tomatis Method, used to enhance listening skills – was consulted. He soon recognized that the fatigue and depression began when the chanting ceased, and he recommended that the chanting – a vital link to creation – be resumed. Within a few months, the monks had regained their vitality and once again were able to perform their duties with only a few hours of sleep.

Tomatis noted that Gregorian chants contain all of the frequencies of the human voice. He concluded that the therapeutic effects of vocal harmonics occur with sounds at about 2000 hertz (Hz), sounds that are created not in the mouth but by the bones of the cranium and skull, and resonate in all of the bones of the body.

Tibetan monks have created a chanting technique, called "toning" or "voice chording," that produces overtones. A monk who has mastered this technique can simultaneously create three notes: a deep bass note called the fundamental, a second note one octave higher, and a third note a fifth higher. In one study, the bass note of a Tibetan monk's chant was found to be 75.5 Hz, two octaves below middle-C. This deep, guttural sound has often been used to invoke the deities. (By comparison, an opera singer's deepest range reaches approximately 150 Hz.) When producing overtone chants, a monk rapidly and continually changes the shape of his larynx. It is this control and consistency that shape the quality of the overtones.

Research has shown that even simple toning immediately produces alpha brain waves, and for this reason it is used by many as a system of healing. When we shape our mouth and repeat vowel sounds, we produce a strong internal vibration that permeates through every cell and helps restore natural harmony among all parts of the body. One can practice toning by voicing the vowel sounds while sitting or standing in a relaxed position, preferably alone. To do so, allow your body to relax and give each tone full expression – which, by the way, may include making the silliest faces. It is the vibration of tone traveling to every part of the body that induces harmony. Through toning, one can become attuned to the "Music of the Spheres."

The Tibetan monks say they seek to make their bones sing, rather than relying entirely on their voices, thus relieving the stress on their throats. How this occurs is explained by Alfred Tomatis: "As the bow sets violin strings vibrating, but it is the violin body which sings, so with proper chanting posture, the larynx of the monks contacts the vertebral column, thereby setting the axial bones to sing."

Thus, in toning, the sounds come not only from the throat, but from deep within us, vibrating from the spine, the skull, and the solar plexus. Air that travels through the larynx and vibrates the vocal cords is transformed into sound waves, which are greatly amplified by resonators such as the oral and nasal cavities, pharynx, chest cavity, and bones. The voice and its resonators are described by Kristin Linklater in her book *Freeing the Natural Voice*:

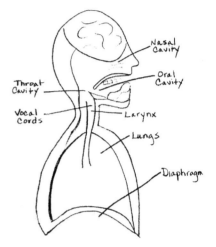

Toning resonators

> The re-sounding of resonating surfaces with the body, available to the initial vibrations of sound, are virtually uncountable considering that bone, cartilage, membrane and muscle can all serve as amplifiers and conductors. The harder the surface, the stronger the resonance: bone is the best, cartilage is very good, and toned-up muscle can provide a good resonating surface, but a flabby, fleshy, unresistant area will only muffle and absorb vibrations (like a heavy velvet or a sponge). The voice finds its most satisfying resonators where there are clearly defined hollows and empty tunnels in the architecture of the body, such as the pharynx, the mouth, the nose; but the bony structure of the chest, the cheekbones, the jawbone, the acoustically powerful sinus hollows, the skull, the cartilage of the larynx and the vertebrae of the spine all contribute to resonance.

Healing with music and sound, as we have described, has been used for thousands of years in all cultures throughout the world. Since the early 20th century, however, the medical profession has largely – but not entirely – ignored this type of healing. Music therapy has found a minor place in modern medicine as means for reducing stress and inducing relaxation.

Music therapy is also useful for emotional and psychological healing, to bring the mind and body back into harmony. Pitch, rhythm, and harmony are the basic elements of music. Music has been used to move us in many ways. It is used in ceremonies and celebrations. It marches soldiers to war, and it is used to celebrate peace. Music soothes a crying soul, lulls a child to sleep. It is found in every culture, past and present. No wonder music has been so effective as a therapeutic tool! Different instruments have different sounds that have distinct effects upon us. There is music to elevate, music to depress. Music to stimulate, music to relax. Music to repress, music to express.

Sound Healing

The effectiveness of sound healing is now being rediscovered. In his book *The Power of Sound*, a treasure for anyone interested in the world of sound, Joshua Leeds writes:

> Be aware of the power of sound; use it consciously.
> As with any substance, there can be positive and negative applications. Consider music and sound as 'thinking people's drugs.' They can enhance, arouse or depress. Like food, water, wine, sex and pharmaceuticals, it all comes down to frequency and dosage. The question becomes: how often and how much? Applied to the effectiveness of auditory stimulation, as well as nervous system balance, the answer is always individual. This is the nature of sound: subtle, powerful, personal.

There are sounds that can drive one to suicide and sounds that can heal. Those suffering from tinnitus (a high-pitched sound in the ears) are known to have ended their lives because of the constant, insufferable sound. People who are sensitive to the 60-Hz hum of electrical transformers may experience nausea, dizziness, and migraine headaches. Currently, a low hum heard by many people in the mountains near Taos, New Mexico, is driving about two percent of the population away every year.

Sound therapy, or soundwork, differs from the use of music as therapy. Whereas music therapy uses melodies and rhythm to induce relaxation and reduce stress, soundwork employs sound or physical vibrations to heal. There is sound within music, of course, but not all sounds are musical. The common element lying within both forms of therapy is vibration and frequency.

Soundwork is the application of specific vibrations that affect the body's nervous system. It utilizes vibration, the principle of resonance, and entrainment. Entrainment can be thought of as forced resonance. A strong rhythm not only activates a resonant rhythm, but also can change a slightly different rhythm to equal it. In the body, entrainment occurs when an external rhythmic stimulus alters and synchronizes the pulses. Physicists define entrainment as a "mutual phase-locking of two oscillators"; for example, pendulums in very close proximity will begin to oscillate in phase.

Sound therapy is neurologically based, sculpting structures and shifting consciousness. It alters physiological responses and affects emotions. Various forms of vocalization, such as toning, chanting, and singing, affect the physiological responses of the body. Studies have shown that these effects include increased oxygenation of the blood and cells, the enhancement of the immune system by increased levels of interleukins and lymphatic circulation, and an increase in endorphins and a decrease in stress hormones such as cortisol.

Soundwork has the specific intention of affecting a patient on a physiological and neurological level. Resonance is the key element in sound healing. Each system in the body, each organ, each cell, has a natural resonant frequency at which it vibrates. When certain vibrations of external origin pass through the body, they affect the parts that have a natural resonance with those specific vibrations. By directly applying sound to living matrix, the nervous system is globally and profoundly affected.

Although some sound therapists use specific tones or directly apply physical vibrations to parts of the body to heal certain conditions, other therapists prefer chanting or using instruments that produce sounds with rich resonances to help restore the body's own harmonic pattern.

Our bodies have two basic electrical systems. One is called the nervous system, and in it electrical currents pass along networks of nerve fibers. The other electrical system, discovered more than 5,000 years ago by the Chinese, has channels called meridians and forms the basis of acupuncture. According to acupuncture theory, the body has patterns of energy, and when the flow of this energy is impeded or disrupted, disharmony and illness will ensue. To restore health, the acupuncturist stimulates the appropriate meridians in order to balance the energy flow to various parts of the body. Recent research has shown that vibrations and sound, as well as acupuncture, can affect the flow of energy along the meridians.

It also has been discovered that the human nervous system responds most strongly to certain intervals between sounds. It is the lack of sound, the space between sounds, that is the determining factor – not the sound itself.

Furthermore, the ears are not the only way that sound reaches the brain. Sound vibrations are transformed into electrical nerve impulses by the ear, and these nerve impulses are sent to the brain. At the same time, sound can cause the temporal bones of the skull to vibrate, which in turn causes vibrations in the fluid surrounding the brain. Inside the skull, the sphenoid bone holds the pituitary gland in a kind of cup or saddle. The vibrations traveling in the fluid cause the "wings" of the sphenoid bone to flap, which stimulates the pituitary gland to secrete hormones that affect the entire body. Thus, sound not only is "heard," but also can stimulate a hormonal response. Physical vibrations that reach the skull can often affect the pituitary gland and cranial nerves.

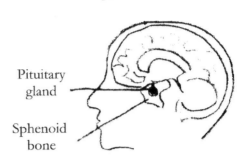

Sphenoid stimulates pituitary

Ten of our 12 cranial nerves lead either directly or indirectly to the ear. The vagus nerve – the longest nerve, also known as "the wanderer" – is directly connected with the ear. This nerve controls many of the autonomic (parasympathetic) functions of our nervous system and is responsible for what are literally our gut reactions. As it wanders from the ear, the nerve next reaches the tongue, larynx, and pharynx, where it supplies partial sensation as well as motor impulses to the vocal cords (the voice of expression). Its next stop is the heart and lungs. It then dips down to the diaphragm and innervates some of the internal organs along with the entire digestive tract, and then communicates with our sacral nerves.

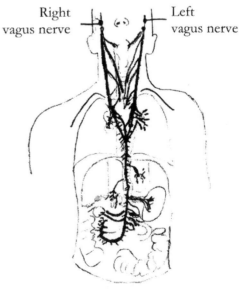

Sound affects vagus nerves

Neurologically and physiologically, sound affects us deeply and completely.

Vibration Therapy

A number of researchers have shown that applying vibrations to specific parts of the body can help the healing process. For instance, some practitioners apply vibrating tuning forks to acupuncture and acupressure points. In my research, I have shown that the vertebral bones respond beautifully to direct stimulation by vibrating musical tuning forks. Tuning forks are a handy means for inducing sympathetic resonance in the body.

The body is a natural resonator, with each organ, tissue, bone, and fluid singing its own song. Sympathetic resonance occurs when one vibrating body induces a harmonic vibration in another body. When we determine what the natural vibration frequencies of the body are, it then will be possible to apply the optimal frequency to any part of the body to restore its natural resonance, and bring the body and spirit into alignment with one another and the natural cosmic cycles.

Sound is a potent tool for transformation. Sound is an essential nutrient that sculpts our nervous system in both the most dramatic and most subtle of ways. Whether using the voice for chanting and toning, or using chimes, gongs, bells, rattles, or drums, or applying physical vibrations with tuning forks or a vibrating table, the effect on the human body can be profound. Healing with sound must always be undertaken with great care and consideration.

The wise healer seeks to restore the body's natural harmony. Plato wrote: "The Muses gave us music to help the soul restore its order and harmony."

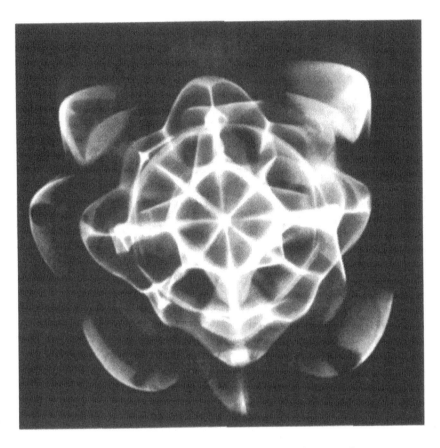

Complex pattern in a vibrating liquid created by a single tone.

— *From* Cymatics: A Study of Wave Phenomena and Vibrations, *by Hans Jenny, © 2001 Macromedia Publishing. Used with permission.*

CHAPTER 3

THE SOUL OF HARMONY AND THE SCIENCE OF HARMONICS

*God made a statue of clay in His own image,
and asked the soul to enter into it: but the soul
refused to be imprisoned, for its nature
is to fly about freely and not to be limited and
bound to any sort of capacity. The soul did not wish
in the least to enter this prison. Then God asked
the angels to play their music, and as the angels played
the soul was moved to ecstasy, in order to make
the music more clear to itself, it entered his body.*
—*Sufi legend*

EVERYTHING WE SEE, hear, smell, taste, and touch – all that we perceive – vibrates. Every atom, cell, tissue, and bone vibrates. Vibrations produce sound, vibrations produce light. It is vibration that produces the brilliance and colors of gems and the sweet sounds of a Beethoven sonata. Not only are we formed of vibrations, but we move and live within them. Whether we can see or hear an object, whether its vibrations are imperceptible or perceptible, the vibrations still exist. It is the speed of the vibrations that enables them to be either visible or audible. Everything we perceive has its sound and its form.

The universe is filled with many vibrations of sound, and inherent in every sound lies harmony. In many ancient cultures, it was believed that highest goal of music is to reveal the essence of the uni-verse – the one song that all music reflects.

Through technological advances, we are now able to gather information from the farthest reaches of space and from the ocean's depths. Though it was once assumed that profound silence prevailed in deep space and the deep sea, we are now discovering the many sounds that can be heard, sounds described as grunting, howling, and crackling.

Sound is energy that vibrates through a medium, and these vibrations are transmitted by a movement of molecules that ripples out in all directions. These ripples are waves that carry forth information. The thinner the medium, the more power sound needs to travel outward. In water, sound travels 4–5 times faster than in air. Since the human body is made up primarily of water, it is an excellent conductor of sound.

Sound is measured objectively by its frequency – the number of vibrations, or cycles, per second. Scientists use the term "hertz" to denote cycles per second. Ten hertz (abbreviated Hz) means 10 cycles per second. We apply the word "sound" to those frequencies our ears can hear. Most of us can hear vibrations between 20 and about 20,000 Hz. For most of us, unfortunately, hearing has already declined by the fourth decade in life to the extent that we are only one-tenth as sensitive to higher-frequency sounds. Common factors that contribute to hearing loss include exposure to intense sounds (noise), head trauma, bacterial infections, and decreased oxygen supply to the brain.

Vibrations above our hearing range are called ultrasonic; those below it are called infrasonic. Some animals, such as bats, crickets, and dogs, can hear in the ultrasonic range, while other animals, such as elephants, communicate in the infrasonic range.

When a string on a musical instrument is plucked or struck, it will vibrate at a specific frequency. For instance, when a middle-C note is played, whether on a piano or a guitar, the string will vibrate at approximately 256 cycles per second, or 256 Hz. If that string is shortened by one-half, it will vibrate at twice the rate, or 512 Hz, and its pitch is higher. If the string is made twice as long, it will vibrate more slowly, at one-half the rate, or 128 Hz, and its pitch is lower.

Pitch and Tone

Pitch is what we experience subjectively. How each of us interprets the frequencies that reach our ears might be different. The pitch of a sound corresponds directly to its frequency. The faster the vibration, the higher the pitch; the slower the vibration, the deeper and lower the pitch.

Tone is also a subjective attribute of sound. Tone gives sound its shape, its color, its dimension. Essentially, tone is the quality we attribute to sounds. Rhythm is a pattern of sound, a beat, like the beating of the heart. Rhythm structures music. Organic life is rhythmic, and rhythm moves the human body.

When we hear a note played on a musical instrument or sung by a voice, it is not just pure, single tones that are heard, but a mixture of tones called partials. The lowest frequency is called the fundamental and the higher frequencies are referred to as overtones. Each overtone is a geometric multiple of the

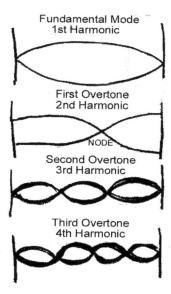

Overtones and harmonics

fundamental. These overtones (harmonics) give beauty and fullness to sound. In his delightful and practical book on vocal harmonics, *Healing Sounds*, Jonathan Goldman wrote, "Harmony is the ratio and the relationship between tones and their rhythmic patterns."

In the 6th century BC, Pythagoras, using a single-stringed instrument called a monochord, developed a theory of musical harmony based on whole-number ratios. Pythagoras believed that by studying the monochord, one could come to know the secrets of the uni-verse (one string, one song). He told his followers that when dealing with harmonic principles, they should ignore their ears, because hearing was prone to variation and error. He wanted them to work primarily with the harmony of numbers.

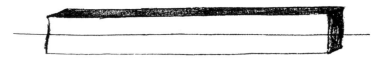

Monochord

Pythagoras related the pitch of a tone to the length of the string that creates that sound. The shorter the string, the higher the note that is created. Instead of using measured lengths, Pythagoras worked out a system using ratios of the lengths, a process that leads to a 12-note scale. That system is still in use today.

To Pythagoras, harmony was created by a numerical ratio that not only occurred in music, but also was an essential component in architecture, and was even perceptible in the heavens. This special ratio – designated phi, and equal to 1.1618... – has been referred to as the Golden Mean, the Golden Ratio, the Golden Section, and the Divine Proportion. The Golden Section is described when a line is cut into two unequal parts such that the ratio of the whole to the larger part is the same as the ratio of the larger part to the smaller one. Much that we perceive as perfect and beautiful in nature and art seems to follow the Golden Ratio. In nature, this beautiful proportion can be found in the shapes of leaves, plants, and nautilus shells, and even in the Earth's interior. It is found in architectural constructions, such as the Greek Parthenon and other beautiful temples. Sound gives structure and beauty, which exists everywhere. Even the human body is proportioned to the Golden Ratio, including the bones of the spine.

In his book *Music, the Brain, and Ecstasy*, Robert Jourdain depicts a correlation between the heavens and each note of the musical scale.

Do	Dominus	God in Humanity
Re	Regina Coeli, Queen of Heaven	The Moon
Mi	Microcosmos, Small Universe	The Earth
Fa	Fatus, Fate	The Planets
So	Sol	The Sun
La	Via Lactae	Milky Way
Si (ti)	Sidereal, Stars	All Galaxies
Do	Dominus	God, Creator, Absolute

Our language is embedded with terms relating to the heavens, even everyday words such as "consider" and "disaster." When we are *considering* something (Lat. sidereus = heavenly) we are conversing with the stars, and *disaster* (Gk. aster = star) befalls us when we go against the stars. Perhaps with *consideration* we can avoid *disasters*.

The Natural Harmony of 12

Although the Western musical scale as we know it today is the result of a mixture of musical traditions that have been arbitrarily simplified, it nonetheless reflects the universal principles that underlie those sequences of sound that the human mind interprets as music. An octave has eight full tones (notes), traditionally depicted as Do, Re, Mi, Fa, So, La, Ti, Do. The eighth tone is a repeat of the first tone but at twice the frequency of the first. An octave also may be divided into 12 semitones.

These 12 divisions of pitch seem to be the right number for our brains to easily distinguish them. Coincidentally, the 12 tones are sufficient to produce music fully rich in their harmonics. The Chinese, Polynesian, and Scottish five-tone scale systems, the Western seven-note diatonic scale, and virtually all of the other major musical scales can be considered subsets of the 12-tone chromatic musical scale.

Researchers at Duke University in North Carolina have found that the 12 tones of an octave very closely match the peaks in the pitch of human speech. They propose that the structure of music is rooted in the characteristics of the human voice. An acoustic analysis of over 100,000 speech samples of English sentences showed that the top 10 frequency peaks matched the intervals used in the 12-octave chromatic musical scale. Analyses of speech in Mandarin, Farsi, and Tamil produced the same correlation. The researchers note that apart from animal calls, speech is about the only natural sound that we hear as tones.

Ethnomusicologists have found that musicians in almost every culture say that tones exactly one octave apart are similar. Octave equivalence appears to be a universal harmonic phenomenon.

It is noteworthy that the number 12 also appears in our designations of time. Day and night are assigned 12 hours each, and there are 12 months in a year. The zodiac consists of 12 signs. Historians point out that such use of the number 12 comes down to us from the ancient Sumerians and Babylonians, but they are unable to tell us why it has persisted for so many thousands of years after the fall of those civilizations. Consider too that the tribes of Israel number 12, as do the apostles. Twelve is the number of the main meridian channel in acupuncture. Even life is particular, in that all Earth life forms selectively take up carbon-12 in preference to the isotope carbon-13. All in all, the number twelve seems to signify a cycle of completion.

The Greeks and others believed that the Pythagorean musical scale had a universal origin, and that sounds trickle down from the heavens. The physical laws that apply to sound are not peculiar to sound; they also regulate the rhythms of the universe. Plato, in his dialog *Timaeus*, wrote that the Pythagorean musical scale reflects the soul of the world.

The mysterious Lambdoma, or Pythagorean Table, relates ratios to musical frequencies. In the 1920s, Hans Kayser, a German scientist, used the Lambdoma to support his theory that the fundamentals of musical harmonics are essentially the same as the principles of the harmonic structure of matter. He believed that the whole-number ratios of musical harmonics correspond to the underlying relationships in the periodic table of elements, and he observed their applications in chemistry, physics, and astronomy as well as in applied techniques such as crystallography and spectroscopy.

The 12 semitones of an octave are not arbitrary; they are indeed a reflection of our bodies' innate harmonic structure. They are built into our bodies, brains, and bones.

Musicologists have found that versions of the Pythagorean musical scale are found in almost every culture throughout the world. In the 22-step scale of some Indian music, for example, harmony is sustained by a hidden 12-step Pythagorean scale. The additional 10 tones are employed for ornamental deviations that waver around the core tones. Indian musicians with absolute pitch have trouble identifying the non-Pythagorean tones, demonstrating that their categorization scheme probably is the same as the Pythagorean.

Chinese music shares a common origin with Indian music, but differs greatly in how it applies the universal musical principles. Chinese music is based on "the cycle of fifths," or a pentatonic (five-note) scale. If you were to play only the black keys on a piano, you would be playing a pentatonic scale.

A cuneiform tablet from 1800 BC contains musical notations alongside what appears to be a hymnal text. Other cuneiform texts from that era contain musical "key numbers" that suggest that ancient Sumerians and Babylonians possessed a coherent musical theory. Reconstruction of this music has revealed that this ancient civilization had a musical scale that is very similar to that developed by Pythagoras.

Physiological Basis of Harmony

For more than 2,000 years after Pythagoras discovered that harmony is determined by small, whole-number ratios, musicians, mathematicians, and philosophers speculated about the meaning of this whole-number phenomenon. It was not until the 1800s that a physiological explanation for whole-number harmony was developed. Hermann Helmholtz (1821–1894), one of the truly great thinkers of that era, undertook a comprehensive analysis of the mechanics of harmony and the physiological processes involved in the perception of harmony and music.

Helmholtz's early studies included the physical cause of harmony and disharmony, the motion of strings on a violin, and the vibration of air in pipes. In his physiological research, he elucidated the mechanics of the small bones of the ear and the acoustical vibrations in the labyrinth of the ear. Helmholtz also published a paper on the Arabic-Persian musical scale and another on musical temperament before completing his opus, *On the Sensations of Tone as Physiological Foundation for the Theory of Music*, in 1862.

Helmholtz found that the whole-number ratios that determine harmony can be explained by how the ear converts sound into nerve impulses. "The ear resolves all complex sounds into pendular oscillations, according to the laws of sympathetic vibration," he wrote, "and it regards as harmonious only such excitements of the nerves that continue without disturbance." To Helmholtz, non-harmonious disturbances are created when the ear receives sounds that are not of the same pitch, resulting in the sensation of disturbing beats.

Furthermore, Helmholtz showed that Pythagoras's numerical relationships could be explained mathematically, using Fourier equations to deal with complex wave phenomena and break them down into their simplest components. When applied to musical harmony, Fourier analysis shows that partial tones must be exactly one, two, three, four, etc., times that of the fundamental tone. These whole numbers determine the harmonic ratios.

Harmony of the Cosmos

When Pythagoras spoke of the "Music of the Spheres," he was not using the expression metaphorically. His disciples believed that he alone among mortal men had heard the music of the spheres. The seven-string lyre was thought to represent the harmony of the spheres. Each string of the lyre represented one of the planets, and the musical sounds themselves were given the names of planets. Because the mathematical laws reflected in the musical scale and the cosmic spheres appeared to be related, music was regarded as a natural connection between the soul and the heavens, between matter and spirit.

Ptolemy, the illustrious Roman astronomer who lived in Alexandria, Egypt, about 150 AD, was so taken with the Pythagorean idea that a planet's orbit correlated with the vibrations of a taut single string that he named his treatise on the mechanics of the cosmos *Harmonia*.

In the early 17th century, Johannes Kepler (1571–1630) came to work in Prague with the renowned Danish astronomer Tycho Brahe. After Brahe died, Kepler took over his position. In 1619, he published *Harmonices Mundi Libri V* – five books about the harmony of the world. Kepler was the first to propose that the orbits of the planets are elliptical and that our solar system possesses a coherent, harmonic structure. One of his most famous works is the Third Law of Planetary Motion, which he called the octave reduction.

It was this law – not an apple – that led Newton to his law of gravitation.

Kepler's discovery of the natural laws of planetary motions gave birth to modern astronomy. But he was more than a great scientist; he was a musician as well. Like the Pythagoreans, he was an ardent seeker of a universal truth, and he believed geometry and music are intricately woven together to form a harmonious and structured universe.

According to Kepler's explanation, God caused the planets to move from their initial circular orbits to elliptical ones because they would produce more beautiful sounds. These elliptical orbits, he claimed, were precisely those that oscillate in the same ratios as the Pythagorean musical scales.

"For this reason," Kepler states, "we should not be surprised that men discovered the beautiful, effective succession of tones in the musical modes when we see that in so doing they did nothing but imitate God's work, thereby playing down to Earth the drama of the celestial motions."

The ancient concept that all music on Earth is only a pale reflection of or substitute for the harmony in heaven seemed to be confirmed by Kepler's finding that the same mathematical ratios are found in both music and the movement of the planets. Long before human music was sounded on Earth, primal music was created in the heavens.

Modern scientists have attempted to create representations of the sounds of the orbiting planets. John Rodgers and Willie Ruff of Yale University created a work titled "A Realization for the Ear of Johannes Kepler's Astronomical Data from Harmonices Mundi" by programming the angular velocities of the planets into a synthesizer using Kepler's data. They assigned a low G to Saturn, and then let Kepler's laws define the tones of the other planets. The sound spectrum of the six visible planets – Mercury, Venus, Earth, Mars,

Jupiter, and Saturn – covers eight octaves. This eight-octave range is close to the range of human hearing.

Both Pythagoras and Kepler saw harmony in the vast structure of the cosmos. But does this harmonic relationship extend to matter at the atomic level? One of the Hermetic laws states, "As above, so below." What this saying implies is that from the orbiting of the planets around the sun to the orbiting of electrons around an atom, the same fundamental tones and their harmonics are created.

Atomic Harmony

Our next exploration takes us into the miniature world of atoms. Niels Bohr, early in the 20th century, developed a model of the atom that had electrons orbiting a nucleus in the same manner that planets orbit the sun. Paul Dirac proposed that the spin of the orbiting electrons had to be either positive or negative with respect to the direction of the electron's orbit, and that the spin was always a whole-number multiple of Planck's constant. Planck's constant, designated as h, has a value of 6.626×10 to the neg. 34th, and is the proportionality that relates the energy of a photon to its frequency. Wolfgang Pauli's exclusion principle states that no two electrons around an atom can have the same spin at the same time. The Pauli exclusion principle was later generalized to the four quantum states (spin, mass, momentum, and position) of the orbiting electrons. This version states that no two electrons can have the same values for all four states.

In the latter part of the 20th century, physicists demonstrated that paired electrons – one with a positive spin and the other with a negative spin – not only "remember" their state when separated, but also seem to be able to "communicate" with one another at a distance. If the spin of one electron is changed, its paired "mate" instantly changes too.

The idea that electrons can store information and then communicate this information has been put forth by Jean E. Charon, a French physicist-philosopher. He wrote: "The electron encloses a space that is able, first, to store information, second, to make this information available again during each pulsation period of its cycle by way of a sort of 'memory system,' and to control complex operations by communicating and cooperating with the other electrons of the system."

Charon thought that the electron is like a miniature "black hole" because of its immense density, and that it exhibits the characteristic curved space and curved time of the traditional black hole. Because an electron is one of the few elementary particles that does not disintegrate, Charon believed that everything stored by the electron can be retrieved in a future cycle. He also believed it is the spin of the electron that stores information, and that this information can be "exchanged" with the help of photons that behave like messengers.

Charon spoke of "memory," "cognition," and "communication" taking place at the level of the electron. Indeed, he saw the electrons as the prime source of stored information. Information between electrons is "communicated" by means of photons. Because of the quantum restrictions that apply to electrons (Pauli's exclusion principle), the communication process takes place in whole-number steps – in a harmonic progression, much like a musical scale. It is as if electrons are communicating their "tones" to one another. Thus, it appears that the harmonic laws of the planets have characteristics that are similar to the laws that apply to orbiting electrons.

The research of Wilfried Kruger, a German musicologist, expanded the work of Charon. Kruger discovered a great correlation between the structures of atoms that sustain life, such as oxygen, nitrogen, carbon, and phosphorus, as well as in RNA and DNA, and the intervals found in a musical scale. He suggested that oxygen, having an atomic number of 8, is the element that represents the octave. He went on to say that the eight electrons and eight protons of the oxygen atom form a major scale in which the positive spin is the full tone and the negative spin is the semitone. Remember that spin is the movement of a body around its own axis and that the spin is always a whole-number ratio – in other words, in harmonic proportions. Kruger went even further, showing a close relationship between the microcosm and the harmonics of music. He explained that the nucleus of the oxygen atom, with its protons, has twelve steps – the precise number of intervals found in the scale formed by the atomic model.

A noted scholar of Tibetan Buddhism, Lama Govinda (1898–1985) poetically depicted a similar idea: "Each atom is constantly singing a song, and each moment this song creates dense or fine forms of greater or lesser materiality."

In modern physics, string theory provides strong support for the idea that vibrations are at the heart of all matter. In his book and TV series titled *The Elegant Universe*, Brian Greene of Columbia University applies the term "strings" to the tiniest bits of matter. Strings are "wiggling strands of unimaginable smallness" that combine to create the subatomic particles that collectively make up atoms. The different ways that strings vibrate, Greene explains, give the subatomic particles their unique properties, such as mass and charge.

It is interesting to note that vibration is what characterizes strings. Just as the vibrations of a single cello string can create different musical notes, the tiny strings that lie at the deepest core of matter vibrate to create different kinds of particles and forms of energy. These oscillations compose a grand cosmic symphony that is the same from the micro scale to the macro. What we perceive as reality is strung together by these squiggly-wiggly strings, connecting us to the many hidden dimensions of this universe.

"*As above, so below.*"

Cellular Harmony

Do harmonic laws apply to living matter as well? Perhaps so. As William Congreve wrote, "Music hath charms to soothe the savage breast, to soften rocks, or bend a knotted oak." Cows produce more milk and chickens lay more eggs when they hear music. Some devoted gardeners believe that plants grow better when bathed in soft music. In one study, Dorothy Retallack grew corn, squash, and flowers in five identical greenhouses. One greenhouse had no music played in it. Each of the other four had one type of music played constantly. The plants in the greenhouses that "listened" to Bach or Indian classical music had the most significant growth – the flowers were more abundant and the squash vines grew toward the loudspeakers. Country/western music seemed to have no effect – the plants grew as much as they did in the greenhouse with no music. Rock and roll music had a negative effect – the plants were smaller and bore far fewer flowers. Other studies in Great Britain, Israel, and the United States have shown by audio spectroscopy that plants and flowers create sounds. A blossoming rose, for instance, creates an organ-like drone.

Although the harmonic vibrations of music are intended for the ear, other parts of a living organism can also respond to these vibrations. Vibrations are sensed by nerves in the skin and can be felt viscerally, and sound travels well along bones. Even on a cellular level, vibrations are felt.

Both cells and elements inside them are capable of vibrating in a dynamic manner, with complex harmonics. Vibrations can cause changes in shape as well as movement and signaling. We know very little about the mechanisms by which vibrational energy is transferred into cells and what kind of harmonic events the vibrations trigger. A great deal of evidence, however, suggests that harmonic vibrations, such as music, can affect the inner workings of a cell. Much research is still needed to identify the frequencies that generate the strongest harmonic responses in cells and tissues, and to learn how to apply those vibrations to promote healing. The study of vibrational frequencies of living organisms is called bioacoustics (literally, "life sounds").

The healing power of the human voice also is being studied. Sharry Edwards, for example, has developed a system for evaluating a person's voice and determining the individual's "signature sound." Each human voice, like a fingerprint, has its own unique patterns. Edwards found that the voices of people with physiological and psychological disorders may have certain frequencies that are abnormal or missing. Her Signature Sounds Works system is designed to provide the necessary feedback to bring the mind/body to a more integrated state by stimulating dormant brainwaves through auditory procedures. She also has demonstrated how low-frequency sound may be used to identify and counter some pathogens in the body.

At the University of California, Los Angeles, Professor Jim Gimzewski is using an atomic-force microscope to measure the vibrations of the surface of a yeast cell. The tiny probe of the microscope is placed on the cell's membrane, where it can detect both the amplitude and the frequency of its vibrations. Gimzewski found that on average, a yeast cell vibrates at 1000 Hz, which is equivalent to the frequency (pitch) of C-sharp to D two octaves above middle-C in the musical scale. He also has studied mammalian cells and has found that bone cells have a lower pitch than yeast cells.

Gimzewski, who previously conducted nanotechnology research at the IBM Zurich Laboratory, calls this technique sonocytology, and he believes that the study of sound produced by individual cells may lead to new diagnostic methods for determining the health of cells. Dead yeast cells emit a low, rumbling sound thought to be generated by random motion of atoms, which the atomic-force probe is sensitive enough to pick up. The frequency of mutated yeast cells is different from that of normal yeast cells, and Grimzewski hopes that sonocytology can be useful in diagnosing cancer, which begins with changes in the genetic expression of cells. It is also possible that this new technique for measuring the vibration of each type of living cell may be used to identify the effects of applied vibration to cells, and to determine the best frequencies to promote and maintain cell health.

When one examines the deeper principles of sound, one taps into the essence and magic of music. As the noted American journalist George Leonard, author of *Silent Pulse*, so eloquently states:

> At the root of all power and motion, there is music and rhythm, the play of patterned frequencies against the matrix of time. More than 2,500 years ago, the philosopher Pythagoras told his followers that a stone is frozen music, an intuition fully validated by modern science; we now know that every particle in the physical universe takes its characteristics from the pitch and pattern and overtones of its particular frequencies, its singing. And the same thing is true of all radiation, all forces great and small, all information. BEFORE WE MAKE MUSIC, MUSIC MAKES US.

CHAPTER 4

SOME MODERN SOUND THERAPIES

Tomatis Method

ONE OF THE MOST SUCCESSFUL and influential sound therapies was developed by Alfred Tomatis, a French physician, who conducted extensive research into the effects of sound on the nervous system. Dr. Tomatis was considered by some of his colleagues to be the Einstein of the ear. He was particularly interested in listening deficiencies, and he developed a method for improving listening skills. Tomatis felt that when a person's listening function is enhanced, the brain's capacity to learn becomes enhanced.

On the basis of his research, Tomatis came to believe that sound is a nutrient for the nervous system, and he proposed that one of the ear's primary functions is to charge the nervous system with electrical impulses generated by sound. The brain, and the neocortex in particular, he said, is energized by certain harmonics, which he called "charging sounds." When the brain is well "charged," a person's ability to concentrate, organize, and remember is greatly enhanced.

The Tomatis Method, which uses music and sound to retrain the listening process, is practiced in more than 250 learning centers throughout Europe and North America. These centers offer a comprehensive medical, psychological, and social treatment for children and adults with learning disabilities, attention deficit disorders, dyslexia, autism, and other sensory or motor skill deficits. The Tomatis Method also has been successful in treating psychological disorders such as depression. Many singers and musicians say that the Tomatis Method has enabled them to fine-tune their listening skills.

Although the ear is the primary means of conveying sound to the brain, sound can also be conveyed to the brain through the skin and by bone conduction. "The whole body hears – the ear is not differentiated skin, but rather skin is differentiated ear," Tomatis said. He also affirmed that bone conduction, particularly through the skull, actually amplifies the sound through resonance.

Tomatis was particularly interested in how sonic vibrations affect the fetus *in utero*. He proposed that the higher-frequency sounds in the mother's speech "nourish" the fetus. He believed that the mother's speech sets the stage for listening skills that are carried into childhood. Tomatis himself was born prematurely, weighing only 3 pounds. He was constantly ill as a child, and he owed his survival to the dedication of a physician who later became a model for Tomatis's lifework.

Tomatis thought that difficult pregnancies can impair or shut down the developing listening process. He sought to expand and develop ways to restore that listening ability, particularly in children. In his view, his method did not so much treat children as awaken the ability within them.

Bio-Tuning and Sonic Induction Therapy

At the Center for Neuroacoustic Research in Encinitas, California (www.neuroacoustic.com), Dr. Jeffrey D. Thompson treats patients with novel sound-healing techniques that he has been developing since 1982. He also offers training workshops for sound-healing practitioners and continues to conduct research to refine the techniques of sound healing and the clinical use of sound.

Like Alfred Tomatis, Thompson conducted research on how sound can directly affect the state of the brain, which in turn brings about changes in the body. He developed a new technique to entrain brainwave activity using binaural beats.

Binaural beats are created by the brain when stereo headphones or speakers are used to present slightly different frequencies below 1000 hertz to each ear. The brain perceives the difference between the frequencies as a beat. To create binaural beats, the difference between the two frequencies should be between 1 and 30 hertz. For example, if the left ear hears 120 hertz and the right ear hears 140 hertz, a beat of 20 hertz is perceived.

Because binaural beats can be created at the same frequencies as our brainwaves, they can be used as an external stimulus to entrain specific neural rhythms by taking advantage of the brain's natural frequency-following response (FFR). Earlier studies have shown that brainwave activity, as measured by the electroencephalograph (EEG), will change to correspond with the fundamental frequency of an auditory stimulus.

Rather than adding separate tones to music to create binaural beats, Dr. Thompson alters the original sound signals in the left and right tracks to create modulated pulses that are perceived as binaural beats. These beats produce a slowing of brainwave activity (i.e., entrainment), which leads to deep relaxation, a lowered heart rate, and reduced stress. He also has developed an "acoustic pacing" system in which stereophonic nature sounds and disguised human body sounds are gradually slowed.

Thompson, a holistic health practitioner, chiropractor, researcher, and musician, began his sound therapy research at his Holistic Health Center in Virginia. After moving to California in 1988, he established the Center for Neuroacoustic Research. In his early work, he investigated the use of sound and used sympathetic resonance as a means of adjusting the vertebrae of the spine. He placed a headphone over a subluxated vertebra and stimulated it with specific sounds. In some instances, the vertebra would move itself back into alignment.

Since developing his unique system for brainwave entrainment, Thompson has devoted his energies to perfecting a sound therapy that he calls Bio-tuning and Sonic Induction. He also has created specific audio programs to help balance the body and mind. More than 40 audio programs have been developed, including deep octaves for deep body vibration; music with brainwave entrainment pulses; multi-layered, nonlinear music for relaxation and stress reduction; 3-D realistic recordings for surrounding body and mind; and primordial sounds from the human body, nature, and deep space to awaken deep levels of the subconscious mind.

In order to deliver sound in the most effective way, Thompson designed a sound table and a sound chair equipped with transducers that act like electronic tuning forks, vibrating at the low-frequency ranges that cause the body to resonate. Music and nature sounds are delivered through headphones. The equipment is used to determine the fundamental healing tone that balances the patient's body and brain. Five brainwave frequencies for healing can then be calculated as octaves of the fundamental healing tone.

A recording of the patient's voice singing the exact fundamental healing tone is used in subsequent sessions to re-establish the patient's primary energy pattern and promote inner healing. The voice tone recording is a key component of the Bio-tuning process because only the patient's own voice can produce the unique set of harmonics and overtones that are characteristic of that person. The vibrations produced by the "voiceprint" are instantly recognized by the body and brain. Following Bio-tuning, when a new balance is achieved, a new voice recording may be necessary.

Bio-tuning requires five sessions, followed by monthly re-testing. In phase two, the Bio-tuning process helps the patient to maximize his or her capabilities and self-empowerment.

BioSonic Repatterning

Dr. John Beaulieu developed BioSonic Repatterning after spending more than 500 hours, over the course of two years, in an anechoic chamber – a completely soundproof, non-echoing room – at New York University. The experience of being in such a chamber is something like being in a sensory deprivation tank. Beaulieu was inspired after reading composer John Cage's account of listening to the sound of one's own nervous system.

In the soundproof room, Beaulieu found that the sound of his own nervous system was familiar. He had encountered it many times while meditating or just before falling asleep. He noticed that the sound of his nervous system would change depending on his mental state. When he was calm, the pitch of the sound was low. When he felt agitated or stressed, the pitch was higher and wavered. Being a musician, he noticed several distinct intervals in the sounds of his nervous system. Bringing two tuning forks into the anechoic chamber, he discovered that his nervous system would quickly realign to the sounds of the forks. His insightful realization was that not only did sound affect the nervous system, but also *the nervous system can be tuned like a musical instrument.*

Dr. Beaulieu is a classically trained pianist, a naturopathic physician, and a polarity therapy practitioner, as well as a composer and counselor. He is author of the book *Music and Sound in the Healing Arts*, and he maintains a website on BioSonic Repatterning (www.biosonics.com).

Tuning forks play in integral role in BioSonic healing. Beaulieu believes that sounds generated by tuning forks are based on sonic ratios that are inherent in nature. When two tuning forks are tapped simultaneously, the combined sound is a pure musical interval. These musical intervals are based on harmonic divisions of the monochord developed by Pythagoras and his followers. These archetypal intervals realign the nervous system and restore the natural rhythms (pulse, breathing, craniosacral) of our body.

BioSonic means "life sound," and Beaulieu views everything in life as vibration. The more aware we become of our own inner vibrations, the more harmonious our inner and outer worlds become. The goal of BioSonic Repatterning is to develop a sonic understanding of the relationship between one's inner self and the external world, to the point where the division becomes nonexistent.

Dr. Beaulieu states that each person has a "life sound" – a fundamental sound. To Pythagoras, the full-length string of the monochord produces the fundamental sound, and each division produces a harmonic sound. Similarly, Beaulieu regards the body's structure and rhythms as harmonics of a fundamental sound. Finding a person's fundamental sound is a process of moving from a vibrational state of dissonance to a state of resonance. Dr. Beaulieu defines dissonance as being out of sonic alignment, a state often felt by an individual as stress. Persistent dissonance creates dysfunction within the vibration of the organs, leading to dis-ease. Beaulieu believes that the role of dissonance is to challenge us to move into different and higher states of energy. If dissonance is largely ignored, it will continue to attract even more dissonance. With awareness and understanding, one is able to move out of dissonance and into a more evolved state of being.

The primary goal of BioSonic Repatterning is to listen with awareness, to come to a place of stillness in which one may access inner senses. Our vibrational environment includes the tone, pitch, and speed of our voice and body movements and "the felt sense pulsation surrounding the communication." Energy is transferred through the voice, and the voice is used to establish resonance. Beaulieu states that with each experience of resonance, we move closer to our source and become "beings of sound mind and body." The natural rhythms of our bodies can be accessed through tuning in and through deep listening.

With practice and experience, it is possible to make your nervous system respond just by thinking of a musical interval. Also, a developed sense of harmonic perception will allow you to "see" what interval another person is tuned into.

Although tuning forks are one of the most powerful tools for healing, BioSonic Repatterning also uses music, toning, chanting, mantras, and other sounds to promote healing and to align a person's natural rhythms. In music, the Golden Mean, or ratio, is known as the fifth. On a piano, starting from C, the fifth note is G – and this C–G interval is referred to as a fifth. Beaulieu believes that in the interval of fifths lies the most potential for healing. He says that "two sounds in relationship create a space for healing." The fifth-interval ratio turns out to be 3:2, and the 3:2 ratio is important on a physiological level. The optimal blood pressure, for example, is 120/80, which is a 3:2 ratio; the optimal sodium/potassium ratio for the body also is 3:2.

New Music composers such as John Cage seek to expand musical concepts and change how people listen to music. Some composers feel that old concepts of harmonics are obsolete. The goal of New Music is to increase awareness, break down mental rigidity, and expand creativity. Beaulieu uses New Music to expand awareness and assist in the integration of consciousness. The key to consciousness listening, says Beaulieu, is flexibility. When we are flexible, we can then truly listen, freely resonate with sound, and *become* sound.

Fabien Maman's Tama-Do

Tama-Do, the Academy of Sound, Color, and Movement, was founded in 1988 by Fabien Maman, a world-famous musician and composer who also has studied acupuncture and vibrational healing. Tama-Do is an international organization with branches in Europe, Russia, China, and the United States. Students of the academy perform healing and harmonizing ceremonies to help bring others into resonance with the cosmos.

Maman has done fundamental research in the field of vibrational medicine. His biological research has demonstrated the beneficial effects of sound on human cancer cells. "The seed of the spiritual is found in the physical," Maman claims. "In the heart of the cells, in the spiral of the DNA is written the divine story. When scientific research, spiritual practice, and artistic expression work together, heaven and Earth are in resonance." In his therapies, Maman uses only elements such as natural sounds, pure colors, and chi movements to nourish the human energy system and help the body restore its balance and health.

By the age of 30, Maman was a successful jazz musician, touring the world with his band. He performed in great concert halls, including Carnegie Hall, the Tokyo Opera, the Paris Olympia, and the Berlin Philharmonic. A composer as well, he received France's Grand Prix de Composition in 1980. While performing in Tokyo, he once asked his hotel to provide a masseur for his band. Instead of a massage therapist, an acupuncturist appeared. Maman was intrigued; it was his first experience with acupuncture. As he watched the acupuncturist work, he realized that it was like music: "He was playing the body like a harp, fine-tuning it with his needles," he observed.

This experience led him on a new journey, studying acupuncture under a master in Paris. Maman's work on the healing power of sound, color, and chi has been the subject of many television and radio shows, and he has given lectures around the world. He has published numerous journal articles and is the author of a book series titled "From Star to Cell: A Sound Structure for the Twenty-First Century," which includes the books *Raising Human Frequencies*; *The Body as a Harp – Sound and Acupuncture*; and *Healing with Sound, Color, and Movement*.

Fabien Maman treats the body on many levels, from subtle energy fields to the physical structure. His approach incorporates the Indian chakras, Chinese chi movements, acupuncture, and Western medicine. After becoming an acupuncturist, he integrated music and acupuncture with his discovery of the sound frequencies of the Shu points. He created his own chi movements called Tao Yin Fa, which correspond with the 12 acupuncture meridians and the Indian chakras.

Maman looks to the spine as the central point of the physical body. The spine is linked to the nervous system, the acupuncture meridians, the chakras, and the endocrine glands. The spine acts a bridge linking together subtle energy fields. Maman found that the spine responds beautifully to tuning forks, and he uses them as a tool for vibrational healing.

Like many other vibrational healers, Maman believes that illness becomes manifest in one's energy field before physical symptoms appear. He believes that emotions and thoughts carry vibrational frequencies that are stored in our auras as either positive or negative energies. Vibrational therapy – combining sound, colors, and chi – can be used to dissolve these negative energies.

Maman went on to show how the color and sound of the human body is harmonically linked to the planets and the stars. Students at Tama-Do perform a harmonizing concert at the change of the seasons with special chi dances. Overtones produced by musical instruments link the participants to the specific star patterns on the night of their performance.

In his vibrational therapy, Maman has created a comprehensive system utilizing non-invasive tools to provide the human energy field with various nutrients. He believes that the use of sound, music, color, and movement allows an individual to move to a more universal consciousness.

Acutonics and Harmonic Medicine

The Acutonics Healing System is a non-invasive, energy-based modality based on Chinese acupuncture and the Indian chakra system. Instead of using needles to stimulate the acupuncture points and chakras, the Acutonics Healing System employs special tuning forks and other sounds to stimulate the body's physical and subtle energy fields. Acutonics offers an integrated and harmonic approach to healthcare based on music, science, Eastern and Western medicine, and metaphysics (www.acutonics.com).

Acutonics and Harmonic Medicine were developed by Donna Carey and Marjorie de Muynck, whose vision created the Kairos Institute in Seattle, Washington. Donna Carey is a licensed acupuncturist, herbalist, and educator. Marjorie de Muynck is a massage practitioner, musician, and composer. Together, they developed a system of harmonic medicine that uses sound to heal.

In addition to precision-calibrated tuning forks, Acutonics employs traditional and modern instruments, including gongs, Tibetan bowls, didgeridoos, drums, rattles, chimes, and sound disks and plates. These instruments help the body to realign with the natural cycle of the cosmos, resulting in balance and spiritual harmony. This harmonic "attunement" eliminates negative patterns at the cellular level. The Acutonics Healing System has been successful in treating a wide range of conditions, such as neurological, respiratory, and gynecological dysfunctions, by restoring psychological, spiritual, and emotional balance.

The Kairos Institute of Sound Healing, operated by Donna Carey, is now located in Llano de San Juan in northern New Mexico. The institute also offers professional training to healthcare practitioners and anyone interested in sound healing. Combining old with new, the Kairos Institute has created a unique blend of instruments and tools for sound healing. The institute's tuning fork products are calibrated to resonate with the body's natural frequencies; higher-frequency tuning forks that correlate with the frequencies of the planets, sun, and moon also are used.

At Kairos, the practitioners' goal is to realign our bodies with the natural cycles of life and the cosmos. It is their passionate belief that sound is the solution.

Holographic Repatterning

Holographic Repatterning was developed by Chloe Wordsworth, a licensed acupuncturist. This comprehensive and dynamic approach integrates old-world systems such as the Indian chakras and Chinese acupuncture with a quantum physics model (www.holographic.org).

Wordsworth has brilliantly synthesized a holistic approach that uses sound, light, color, movement, breath, and touch to transform unwanted negative patterns, using muscle testing as a biofeedback tool. The intention of this work is to enhance our evolution and embody life-enhancing attitudes using the concept of coherence and principle of resonance. When a negative pattern is clearly identified, it can be changed when we are resonating with our innate wisdom.

As a student of Holographic Repatterning, I have continuously been amazed at the instantaneous transformation that can occur with this comprehensive and supportive process.

Vocal Harmonics

Jonathan Goldman is a pioneer in the field of healing harmonics and the use of the human voice as a tool for healing and transformation. In his delightful and practical book *Healing Sounds – The Power of Harmonics*, he describes the transformational power of sound, and explains why the voice is the most suitable instrument for healing and transformation. Goldman examines the science of harmonics (overtones) and its use in sacred practices, with a closer look at the vocal harmonics of the Tibetans, Mongolians, and Tuvans. He goes on to describe new ways of producing vocal harmonics that he has developed and that are relatively easy to learn. Goldman is a master of vocal harmonics and is one of the few people in the Western world to have mastered the art of deep throat singing. He has studied overtone chanting with chant masters of Tibet.

Goldman's ideas and book have struck a chord with me and with many other practitioners of vibrational medicine. The author has been invited to conduct sound healing seminars around the world. Once a year, Goldman holds an intensive healing sounds workshop in the Colorado mountains. He is the director of the Sound Healers Association, based in Boulder, Colorado, a nonprofit educational organization dedicated to research and to promoting awareness of the uses of sound and music as therapeutic and transformational modalities. It offers workshops, seminars, and a correspondence course.

I have had the privilege of learning from Jonathan Goldman at his nine-day "Healing Sounds Intensive," which is held in the beautiful foothills of the Rocky Mountains. In that environment, the celebration of sounds and dance and sacred chants moved me to my core. The feeling of being nurtured by sound filled me with joy and laughter. The experience gave me a much deeper insight and a profound sense of what it means to use the power of sound to transform and heal. For this I am deeply grateful for the teachings of Jonathan, his wife Andi, and their teacher, Sarah Benson.

Vocal harmonics can create changes in our physiology, such as slowing down our heartbeat and respiration, changing brain wave patterns, and releasing certain neurotransmitters and hormones to facilitate altered states. In healing, vocal harmonics is being used to shift energy patterns and remove "stuck" energy.

Goldman stresses that intent is a key factor when using the voice, or other instruments, to heal. It is through the voice that intention can be focused. Goldman has come up with a beautiful, essential, and simple formula: *Frequency + Intention = Healing*. Frequency is the sound used, intent is the energy and consciousness encoded into the sound, and healing is the attaining of a healthy resonance. The formula and how sound can be used to change one's vibratory rate are more fully discussed in his book, *Shifting Frequencies*. But I think that for healing to occur, the participant/patient must be flexible and receptive. It is within this receptive state that healing takes place.

CHAPTER 5

SOUND CREATES FORM

OUR BODIES ARE BATHED IN and surrounded by vibrations. The vibrations that we can see are called light. At higher frequencies are x-rays and gamma rays, which are more energetic and penetrating than light but invisible to us. Radio waves occupy lower frequencies and also are invisible. All that we perceive as being solid actually is made up of vibrating atoms. Atoms in turn are made up of rapidly vibrating subatomic entities, which can be regarded as either particles or waves (vibrations). Not only is matter made up of vibrations, energy is as well. Heat is vibration, light is vibration, electricity is vibration, radio waves are vibration, and so are other forms of energy. Thus, from the point of view of a physicist, the universe as we know it is made up of vibrations.

The air around us is filled with vibrations. When the rate of vibration is within a certain range, our ears can detect these vibrations and convert them into sound. In other words, vibrations that we can hear are what we call sound. Our range of hearing typically is from about 20 to 20,000 hertz (cycles per second). We also can feel vibrations with our skin, our teeth, and our bones; in fact, we can detect a wider range of vibrations by feel than by hearing.

Sound is created by a pulse, a force or burst of energy. It is this burst of energy that causes movement, which in turn causes a compression and then expansion of the atoms and molecules in the immediate vicinity. The compression-expansion is transferred to adjoining atoms and molecules, creating a wave motion that travels away from the originating pulse. Although the wave travels away, the atoms and molecules that transmit the wave remain in their original locations after they have transferred the energy from the pulse. What we hear or feel as vibrations are these waves traveling away from the energy pulse or its source.

Sound Sculpts Shape

The pulse that generates a wave determines its strength and shape. The strength, or volume, of a sound wave is measured in decibels. It is the form or shape of the wave that determines the quality of the sound. The form not only is three-dimensional, but also changes over time, becoming less distinct as the energy of the wave is absorbed by the atoms and molecules that are transmitting it. Because air is transparent, we cannot see the form or shape of a sound with our eyes, the way we can see a wave in water. But our ears are able to "see" the form of sound waves and translate it into nerve signals.

Perhaps in the future there will be computer programs that can calculate and "visualize" the form of a sound wave as it propagates through the air. Scientists already are using supercomputers to create visualizations of how light waves are altered as they pass through different air densities in the atmosphere.

Fortunately, we do not need a supercomputer to visualize the form and shape of sound. That was achieved more than 200 years ago by an ingenious German scientist, Ernst Chladni, who is called the father of acoustic research because of his work in the mathematics of sound waves. In 1787, Chladni published his discoveries in a book, *Entdeckungen uber die Theorie des Klanges* (Discoveries about the Theory of Sound).

Chladni, a musician, filled organ pipes with different gases and then determined the velocity of sound in a particular gas from the pitch produced. But he is best known today for Chladni plates. In his experiments Chladni found that if he placed sand on a metal plate

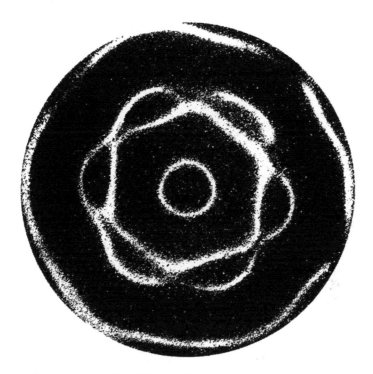

A harmonic pattern produced by speaking into an acoustic tonoscope. The vibrations of the voice are conveyed directly to sand spread on a taut, thin rubber membrane.

— *From* Cymatics: A Study of Wave Phenomena and Vibrations, *by Hans Jenny, © 2001 Macromedia Publishing. Used with permission.*

and then drew a violin bow across the plate at a vertical right angle, the bow created vibrations in the plate that caused the sand to form geometric patterns. Chladni plates have become a popular feature at science museums; using them, children can create symmetrical shapes and beautiful patterns, now referred to as Chladni figures, by running a bow across a metal plate.

A century and a half after Chladni's original work, Dr. Hans Jenny in Switzerland became so intrigued by Chladni figures that he spent 14 years experimenting with powders, pastes, and liquids and photographing the forms that were created by sound. The multi-talented Dr. Jenny was what we would call a Renaissance man —

a family physician, philosopher, scientific researcher, world lecturer, painter, and pianist. He was a student of Rudolf Steiner's method of attaining an inner harmony, called Anthroposophy. Steiner profoundly influenced Jenny's life, and Jenny was such an admirer of Steiner's philosophy that he taught for four years at the Rudolf Steiner school after obtaining his medical degree.

Instead of using a violin bow, Jenny used a frequency generator and loudspeakers or sound transducers to cause the Chladni plates to vibrate. With this equipment, he could vary the frequency (pitch) and the strength (amplitude) of the sound. The results were astounding. Jenny found that sound could create not only symmetrical patterns but also flowing, dynamic shapes that resembled those found in nature. The moving patterns on the vibrating plates appeared to mimic biological, geological, astrophysical, and atomic events. Some patterns, for instance, looked like amoebae fusing or flowers blossoming, while others looked like rotating spiral galaxies or solar flares and sunspots.

Jenny worked with a variety of substances, including sand, lycopodium (club moss spores), metal filings, semi-liquid pastes, and liquids such as water, turpentine, and glycerin. When placed on the disk, the material would start as a formless blob. As vibrations were applied to the disk, the blob would begin to change and move, forming patterns and shapes that appeared to be animated, as if dancing with a life of their own. As the frequency or intensity of the vibration was changed, new patterns would emerge. And when the sound was cut off, the material once again returned to its original formless state.

Hans Jenny had demonstrated that sound is capable not only of moving but also of shaping matter. He took thousands of photographs of the different kinds of shapes and flowing patterns that were created by sound, and he carefully documented his work so it could be replicated by others. Jenny came to the conclusion that all natural phenomena were ultimately determined by their frequencies of vibration. He named his study of wave phenomena

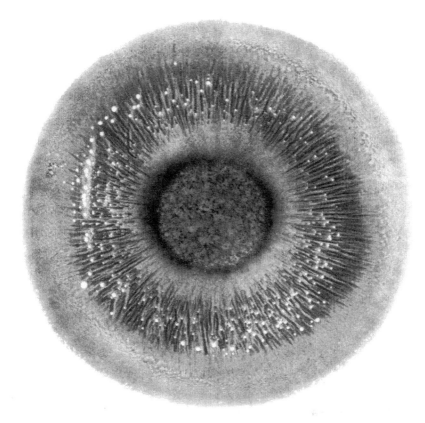

Lycopodium (spores of club moss) on a diaphragm excited by a tone form small round shapes, which dance and unite into organized patterns. As the amplitude of the vibration is increased, spores migrate in radial paths to and from the center, creating an eye-like image.

— *From* Cymatics: A Study of Wave Phenomena and Vibrations, by Hans Jenny, © 2001 Macromedia Publishing. *Used with permission.*

"cymatics," and he published a bilingual book, *Kymatics/Cymatics*, in 1967, followed by a second book, *Cymatics Vol. II*, in 1972.

Cymatics has been applied to healing by Dr. Peter Guy Manners, a British osteopath, who previously found that applying ultrasonic waves to acupuncture points improved healing in certain cases. Manners developed a cymatics device that electronically generates

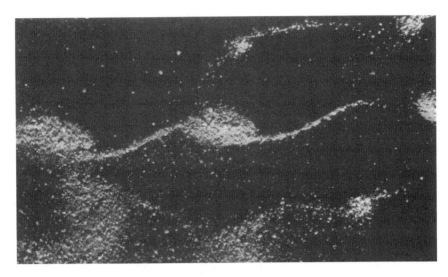

Rotational patterns that look like spiral galaxies are formed by flowing sand stimulated by vibrations from crystal oscillators.

— *From* Cymatics: A Study of Wave Phenomena and Vibrations, *by Hans Jenny, © 2001 Macromedia Publishing. Used with permission.*

specific frequencies for different organs and for diseases caused by imbalance. For more information, visit the websites cymatics.org.uk and cymaticsource.com.

Standing Wave and Resonance

The shapes and patterns created by sound on Chladni plates are the result of what physicists call a standing wave. When sound waves of the same frequency in a fixed space, such as a Chladni plate or a musical instrument, are reflected from the boundaries, the reflected waves are superimposed on the original waves, and the interaction creates an interference pattern that is referred to as a standing wave.

The uniqueness of the sound of a musical instrument is the result of these standing-wave vibrations. It is combinations of standing waves that give different musical instruments their signature sounds. That explains why all violins sound like violins and not like cellos or clarinets. Furthermore, every violin has its own characteristic sounds.

The shape of the spine, after the spinal curves have developed, looks like a simple standing wave. When viewed from the side, a newborn baby's spine has only one curve, known as the primary or kyphotic curve. The secondary, or lordotic, curves begin to develop when the baby is able to sit and learns to crawl, stand, and walk. The primary curve (thoracic) consists of 12 vertebral bones. Together, the two secondary curves (neck and lower back) also have a total of 12 vertebral bones.

Like the other bones of the body, the vertebrae are excellent acoustic resonators. Because each vertebra has its own mass, shape, and size, it can be expected to have a fundamental frequency at which it resonates. The natural resonance of the vertebrae can be used for healing. If the resonant frequency of a particular vertebra can be determined, then it may be possible to restore a subluxated vertebra's natural frequency by using sympathetic vibrations.

The law of resonance states that anything that vibrates reacts sympathetically to its harmonic vibrations. Sympathetic vibration occurs when two objects have the same or very similar resonant frequency. For example, when two violins are placed side by side, and a string on one violin is plucked, the corresponding string on the other violin begins to vibrate. That phenomenon is called sympathetic vibration, or resonance. The effect is much easier to demonstrate with two identical tuning forks, say middle-C (256 Hz). When one tuning fork is struck and begins to vibrate, the second tuning fork spontaneously begins to vibrate. Or if the tuning fork is held near a piano, and the middle-C key on the piano is played, the tuning fork also begins to emit a middle-C sound.

The word "resonance" comes from the Latin *resonantia*, which means to echo, return to sound. Objects that are resonators have the ability to both transmit and respond to their resonant frequencies.

According to a recent study conducted by Clinton Rubin, a biomedical engineer, regular doses of gentle vibrations increased bone density in test animals. Researchers measured the bone density of the hind legs of two groups of sheep. One group then stood on a vibrating platform for 20 minutes a day, five days a week, for one year. A control group of sheep that shared the same pasture did not stand on the vibrating platform. At the end of the year, the bone density of the sheep treated with vibrations was found to be 34 percent greater than that of the control animals. Rubin is now conducting clinical trials with human subjects who have bone-wasting disorders.

Many of the body's harmonic frequencies have yet to be discovered. Given that EEGs and EKGs are measured using relatively simple electronic instruments, one can only imagine the subtle harmonics and rhythms that could be uncovered with the use of more sensitive and complex detection devices.

As it turns out, tuning forks are an effective tool for both testing the harmonic frequency of a vertebra and restoring the vertebra's natural harmonic frequency. In order to find the harmonic resonance of a specific vertebra it is necessary to test a full range of tuning forks on it. At present, my research has determined what seems to be the optimal frequencies for all 24 vertebrae. These resonant frequencies can be used as an adjunct to hands-on adjustments for correcting vertebral subluxations (partial displacement of vertebrae). Placing the correct resonant tuning fork against a vertebra will induce a sympathetic vibration in that vertebra.

When a subluxation is present and a tuning fork with the right frequency is applied to the subluxated vertebra, the bone resets its natural tone. When the vertebra is resonating to its optimal frequency, the surrounding muscles respond with a relaxation that helps to correct the subluxation. In addition, harmonic waves are reverberated throughout the spine, creating coherent harmonic messages that are transmitted through the central and autonomic nervous systems. These harmonic waves help to balance that system, which controls the breath, heart rate, digestion, and other physiological activities. In other words, the vibrations re-tune the nervous system.

The spine is perfectly structured anatomically to produce these harmonic waves. There is evidence that a healthy spine can generate its own harmonic waves to meet the neurophysiological demands of a task at hand. Standing waves that exist between the vertebrae and the heart and brain have a direct impact on the degree and extent of spinal neural integrity. Dis-harmony and dis-ease disrupt the body's inherent harmony, and one way to restore the body's balance is the judicious application of vibrations.

Resonance and sympathetic vibrations affect us deeply in many ways, and they can serve as an instrument of devastation as well as a tool for transformation. In a well-known incident in 1940, for example, the wind's resonance frequency happened to match that of the Tacoma Narrows suspension bridge in Washington state. As a result, the entire bridge began to vibrate and undulate until eventually the bridge shattered and fell apart. And consider a Biblical example of the devastating power of sound: the walls of Jericho came crashing down with just the blow of trumpets!

In his book *The Chiropractor's Adjuster – The Text-Book of the Science, Art and Philosophy of Chiropractic*, David Daniel Palmer, the father of chiropractic, expressed his belief that chiropractic is founded on tone. Did he intuitively know that the bones of the spine are shaped by sound, and that tone is the foundation of a healthy spine? I believe that harmony resounds in our bones, and our bones propagate harmony to our nervous system.

Trager – A Dance, A Song

There is a way of being
which is lighter
which is freer
A way in which work
as well as play
becomes a dance
and living a song
we can learn

—Milton Trager, MD

CHAPTER 6

BONE TONING

BONE TONING IS THE APPLICATION of specific frequencies to the vertebrae in order to generate sympathetic resonances that release the embedded harmonics that lie within the spine.

I began to view the spine as a standing wave when I was attending chiropractic school. At first, I wasn't sure what to make of this concept. Later, when I touched a spine, it "sang to me." It is my training in the Trager® Approach that has given me a greater and more subtle awareness of the rhythm in our bodies.

Standing wave

The Trager Approach was developed by Milton Trager, M.D., who successfully treated challenging conditions such as polio, muscular dystrophy, and Parkinson's, as well chronic pain, stroke, paralysis, and whiplash.

Before a Trager session, the practitioner enters a calm, deep, meditative, all-accepting, all-loving state called "hook-up." In this state of "hook-up" the Trager practitioner resonates with the life-giving force that surrounds and bathes us. This life-giving force is known by many names, such as God, the Great Spirit, or chi energy.

During a session, the client, comfortably dressed, lies on a table. The practitioner gently moves the client's limbs and body using wave-like, rhythmic motions, which tap into the client's natural rhythm. These waves send continuous and repetitive messages that penetrate to the core of the client's body and mind, imparting a feeling of pleasantness and safety. Trager Work gently and lovingly suggests to the client's mind and tissues another possibility, a new way of being. In turn, messages are transmitted from the mind to the body. These signals break up habitual patterns of tension and replace them with new sensations of lightness, freeness, and softness. During a Trager session, tense tissue turns into taffy.

While giving a Trager session, the practitioner also receives one. During a session the practitioner is silently questioning, listening, pausing, sculpting, and questioning again – what is softer, what is freer, what is lighter?

Like homeopathy, the Trager Approach uses less to achieve more. When a practitioner feels resistance from the client's body, the practitioner's movements become even lighter, even softer. Pain should not be experienced by the client during a session, nor tension felt by the practitioner. As the session ends, the client is asked to recall the feeling of freeness. After the session, the client is shown how to return to the light, tension-free state.

Mentastics® is a term coined by the late Milton Trager and his wife, Emily, to describe a form of mental gymnastics, movements directed by the mind to the tissues, which are dumb.

Mentastics is Trager Work off the table. Mentastics can be done lying down, sitting, standing, or walking. It can be done at home or at work. It differs from exercise in that it is not a form or technique, nor are there any time constraints. When doing Mentastics, you can take as much or as little time as necessary to recall the sensations of lightness, softness, expansion, and elongation.

I have been practicing the Trager Approach for almost 20 years, and each session brings renewed awareness of how light, how free and soft we can be. By inducing wave-like motions in the body, Trager Work sets up a harmonic resonance, resulting in standing waves. These standing waves vibrate at the body's most natural frequency, thus allowing for optimal energy transfer and "hook-up." Many other kinds of vibrational medicine, including acupuncture, craniosacral, and homeopathy, also rely on the therapist's ability to "tune into" the client's natural rhythms.

After years of clinical practice as a chiropractor, I began to wonder if each vertebra had a specific tone to which it would respond. The idea of using tuning forks arose out of my background in music and experience with Holographic Repatterning. Tuning forks are not a new tool, by any means. Tuning forks made of stone were used thousands of years ago in Egypt. At the Abu Simbel site, a mural depicts Osiris holding a long rod with an angled tuning fork at the top. The angled piece permits vibrations to enter and run up the spine. The tuning-fork rod is believed to be a tool of resurrection.

The modern metal tuning fork was designed about 400 years ago by a trumpet player named John Score. In music, the most common use for tuning forks is to tune guitars and pianos. In vibrational medicine, many practitioners use tuning forks very effectively in healing sessions.

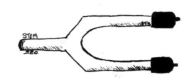

Tuning fork

Developed by Chloe Wordsworth, Holographic Repatterning is an approach to healing that uses modalities such as light, movement, breath, and sound – and it includes the use of tuning forks. It is one of the most comprehensive and dynamic approaches for transforming undesirable thoughts and patterns by changing the frequencies within our system. Holographic Repatterning uses tuning forks to achieve harmonic resonance within the body, bringing harmony to the organs and bones. In the repatterning process, resonance is the key to transforming unwanted patterns, whether they are conscious or unconscious. Once a problem area has been identified, it can then be changed.

One of Holographic Repatterning's main missions is to help the client resonate with life-enhancing attitudes and behaviors.

The human spine consists of 24 movable vertebrae, running in a column from the skull to the sacrum. The spine of a newborn baby has only one primary curve – a kyphotic curve – that allowed him to curl forward to fit in the womb. As the child begins to crawl, sit, and walk, two secondary or lordotic curves develop in the neck and lower back, curving backwards to balance or counteract the forward curve of the upper and mid-back. The normal spine of a walking child has a kyphotic curve that consists of 12 vertebrae (upper and mid-back), and two lordotic curves comprising the other 12 vertebrae (seven cervical/neck and five lumbar/lower back).

With its kyphotic and lordotic curves, the spine looks very much like a standing wave. These spinal curves are essential to the health and flexibility of the spine. Without them, movement and stability would be a much greater challenge. In a standing wave, energy is transferred between the primary wave and its reflection. This suggests that vibrations in the primary and secondary curves of the spine interact and echo off each other to form a standing wave, which helps to maintain the structural and neural integrity of the spine and nervous system.

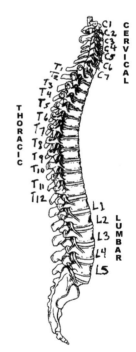

Lateral view of the spine showing kyphotic (backward) curve of the thoracic vertebrae (T1 through T12) and the lordotic (forward) curves of the cervical (C1 through C7 and lumbar (L1 through L5) vertebrae.

When our bones lose their tones because of such factors as trauma, poor nutrition, pathogens, and degeneration, the result in the spine is called a subluxation, or a partial displacement of a vertebra in relation to the vertebrae above and below. This displacement affects the biomechanics of the spine, the vascular system, the nervous system, the surrounding tissues, and the end organ or muscle supplied by that particular nerve.

When the tones of the bones are diminished, a lessening or exaggeration of the spinal curves may result. When these curves become distorted, information cannot be properly transmitted throughout the nervous system, and the stability and flexibility of the spine become compromised.

Search for the Right Notes

During my research, I considered trying to match the individual vertebrae to individual notes of a musical octave. But an octave consists of eight full tones, and I thought it unlikely there would be a one-to-one correspondence between the eight musical tones (with the eighth tone reflecting the first tone but at double the frequency) and the 24 vertebrae. Then one day, Cliff, a 75-year-old musician, was on my chiropractic table, and I told him about my effort to find the tones to which vertebrae might respond. "I feel that the bones of the spine are somehow related to an octave," I said, " but there are twelve bones in each spinal curve and there are only eight tones in an octave."

Cliff's reply was succinct: "You haven't included the five black keys." My spirits soared and my body leaped. That was the missing piece. Now I had an octave of 12 semitones to correlate with the 12 vertebrae in each spinal curve.

My next challenge was how to determine the effect of a vibrating tuning fork on each vertebra. Fortunately, there was a technique available, and one that I was familiar with because of my training as a chiropractor and my work with Holographic Repatterning. The technique is usually referred to as "muscle testing," but the formal

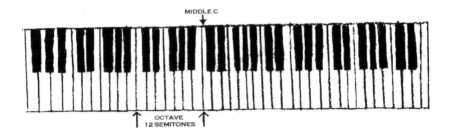

Piano keyboard and octave

term is "applied kinesiology." In Holographic Repatterning, muscle testing is used as a biofeedback tool.

"Muscle testing" is somewhat of a misnomer, since the test actually deals with how the nervous system controls muscle function. The term is a holdover from the time when the test was used to measure muscle weakness in polio patients. Today the test is rarely used to determine whether muscles are strong or weak. Applied kinesiology has developed into a system that uses manual muscle testing to evaluate how the body reacts to various stimuli applied to the nervous system. Applied kinesiology also is known as functional neurology – the study of how the nervous system controls muscle and body functions.

Muscle testing can be applied to any limb, but the arm is most commonly used. The patient holds out an arm and is told to resist downward pressure being applied by the examiner's hand. As the examiner increases pressure, the patient's nervous system locks the muscle, and the muscle is said to test "strong." The examiner repeats the test several times in order to determine the muscle's overall tone and strength. Next the examiner touches, or has the patient touch, a part of the body that is suspected to be malfunctioning. The arm test is repeated, and if there is no malfunction, the test result will again be strong. But if there is a malfunction in that area, then the patient's arm will suddenly weaken and drop. This weak test is repeated several times, alternating with the strong test.

Muscle testing works not only through touching parts of the body, but also when the person being tested holds a substance such as food or a medicine. For instance, muscle testing can be used to find out if a person is allergic to certain foods. It also can be used to determine what vitamins, herbs, or supplements that individual needs. Muscle testing works even when the person being tested does not know what substance is being tested.

Because each vertebra is different in size, shape, and mass, each can be expected to vibrate at its own natural, or fundamental, frequency. Some researchers have reported that the ratio of the weight of the individual vertebrae to that of the spine corresponds to the musical scale. In the hope of verifying such a correlation, I weighed several dry spines but did not find any indication that the weights corresponded to the frequencies of the notes in the musical scale. Future work may find such a correspondence, particularly if vertebrae from young people are weighed before and after they are dried.

I began testing each vertebra with a set of 12 tuning forks that represented one full octave, the 12 semitones from C to B. The corresponding frequencies range from 130.81 Hz to 233.08 Hz.

In order to make a clear sound with a tuning fork, one holds it by the stem and taps it firmly but not hard, preferably against something rubber (rather than on the knee). The fork is held at a slight angle when it is being struck, with the fingers and wrist relaxed. All the action is in the wrist. A second tap is sometimes necessary to create a sustained tone. The vibrations from a single tap last about 20 to 30 seconds. I prefer steel tuning forks to aluminum ones because steel produces a more subtle, purer tone. Aluminum forks, however, are lighter and seem to vibrate for a slightly longer period of time.

Throughout my initial studies, one researcher performed the muscle test on a subject while a second researcher pressed a vibrating tuning fork to one vertebra on bare skin. Each of the 12 tuning forks was applied, one at a time, to each of the 24 vertebrae.

Neither the researcher performing the muscle test nor the subject was aware of which tuning fork was being applied to a vertebra. In many cases, the muscle tester was unaware of which vertebra was being tested.

The testing revealed that, indeed, each vertebra had a preferred frequency. Only one tuning fork out of the 12 produced a strong, positive muscle test response in each of the vertebrae; the other 11 tuning forks produced negative, weak muscle responses. For instance, the atlas (the uppermost vertebra) has a strong muscle test response only when the frequency of the tuning fork is 130.81 Hz. All the other tuning forks elicited a weak, or negative, muscle response.

The Notes of the Spine

It appeared not to matter what part of the vertebra the tuning fork touched, but it was essential that the tuning fork be held directly over the bone. Another important factor was the amount of tissue overlying the bone. Tissue has dampening effect on the vibrations, so the tuning fork had to be applied for a slightly longer period of time when there was padding over the bone. The additional time allowed the bone to "recognize" its optimal frequency.

My research with tuning forks has shown that the 12 bones of each spinal curve are in direct relation with the 12 semitones of an octave – specifically, the first octave below middle-C, with a frequency range of 130.81 Hz to 233.08 Hz.

To find out if the vertebrae were responding to a tone or note rather than a specific frequency, I tested the first cervical and first thoracic vertebrae, which had responded strongly to the 130.81-Hz C tone, with two higher pitches of C – middle-C on the piano (approximately 256 Hz) and an octave above middle-C (512 Hz). Several hundred subjects were tested in this way with the higher pitch notes, and in almost every test, both higher pitches of the note C produced weak muscle responses. These results suggest it was not just the tone that the vertebrae responded to, but also the specific frequency.

The results of my work over many years are summarized in this table:

Cervical Spine

C1 (Atlas)	130.81 Hz (C)
C2 (Axis)	146.83 Hz (D)
C3	164.81 Hz (E)
C4	174.61 Hz (F)
C5	196.00 Hz (G)
C6	220.20 Hz (A)
C7	246.94 Hz (B)

Thoracic Spine

T1	130.81 Hz (C)
T2	146.83 Hz (D)
T3	164.81 Hz (E)
T4	174.61 Hz (F)
T5	196.00 Hz (G)
T6	220.20 Hz (A)
T7	246.94 Hz (B)
T8	138.57 Hz (C#)
T9	155.56 Hz (D#)
T10	185.00 Hz (F#)
T11	207.65 Hz (G#)
T12	233.08 Hz (A#)

Lumbar Spine

L1	138.57 Hz (C#)
L2	155.56 Hz (D#)
L3	185.00 Hz (F#)
L4	207.65 Hz (G#)
L5	233.08 Hz (A#)

In both the cervical spine and the thoracic spine, the first vertebra resonates at the frequency of 130.81 Hz – the C below middle-C.

In each case, the next vertebra resonates with D, the next note in the octave, and so on until B, the seventh note of the octave, is reached at the seventh vertebra. The remaining five vertebrae of the thoracic spine resonate with the five black keys of the octave (C# to A#). The five vertebrae of the lumbar spine also resonate with the five black keys, completing the octave that began with the cervical spine. In the course of my research over the past seven years, tuning forks have been used to test the spines of almost 3,000 persons, and the results have been remarkably consistent, even when the examiner performing the muscle test did not know which vertebra was being tested or which tuning fork was being used. Also, when other chiropractors did the testing, the results were quite consistent, which gives me confidence that the frequencies listed above are specifically "recognized" by their corresponding vertebrae.

Let me note, however, that these frequencies are not absolute. In fact, I have found that they may vary somewhat. Using muscle tests, it appears that the effective frequencies may be as much as 4 or 5 Hz less than those I found with the tuning forks. In the future, more exact data will likely be obtained from the use of a tunable electronic instrument in place of a simple tuning fork.

Modern tuning forks are based on an international standard in which middle-A is defined as 440 Hz. However, since the 1700s the standard for middle-A in Europe varied from about 415 Hz to as high as 455 Hz. This change in pitch was comprehensively chronicled by Hermann Helmholtz in his great classic, *On the Sensations of Tone*. The modern 440-Hz standard was introduced by Johann Sebastian Bach. An alternative was put forward by Giuseppe Verdi, who preferred using 432 Hz as the standard pitch for middle-A. Italy even enacted a law requiring state-supported concert halls to be tuned to the Verdi pitch. The Paris Academy fixed the French pitch for middle-A at 435 Hz. Because of the variation in standard pitch over the past few centuries, it is my feeling that our bodies have learned to recognize a small range of frequencies that produce harmonic resonance.

Song of the Spine

C1 130.81Hz
C2 146.83Hz
C3 164.81Hz
C4 174.61Hz
C5 196.00Hz
C6 220.20Hz
C7 246.94Hz
T1 130.81Hz
T2 146.83Hz
T3 164.81Hz
T4 174.61Hz
T5 196.00Hz
T6 220.2Hz
T7 246.94Hz
T8 138.57Hz
T9 155.56Hz
T10 185.00Hz
T11 207.65Hz
T12 233.08Hz
L1 138.57Hz
L2 155.56Hz
L3 185.00Hz
L4 207.65Hz
L5 233.08Hz

Frequencies of the vertebrae

Toning Subluxations

Bone toning with tuning forks can be used to correct a spinal subluxation. A subluxation is a partial dislocation in which a vertebra is misaligned in relation to the vertebrae above and below. The subluxation adversely affects the biomechanics of joints, local tissues, nerves, the blood supply, muscles, and end organs. When a subluxation is corrected, there is increased blood and nerve supply to local tissues, muscle tone increases, proper biomechanics are restored to the joints, and a balancing of the central and the autonomic nervous systems occurs.

The founder of chiropractic, Daniel David Palmer, proposed that pressure on a nerve results in an increase in the tension of the nerve, which in turn causes an accelerated rate of nerve impulses. In his book *The Chiropractor's Adjuster – The Text-Book of the Science, Art and Philosophy of Chiropractic*, Palmer wrote:

> The amount of nerve tension determines health or disease. In health there is normal tension, known as tone, the normal activity, strength and excitability of the various organs and functions as observed in a state of health. The kind of disease depends upon what nerves are too tense or too slack. Functions performed in a normal manner and amount result in health. Diseases are conditions resulting from either an excess or deficiency of functioning.

Palmer believed that the pressure put on a nerve by a subluxation (stretched, compressed, or inflamed) alters the vibrational frequency of neural transmission, increasing it or decreasing it. An increased rate of neural transmission is the cause of the elevated heat and inflammation that often are found in the subluxated nerve and in the tissues and organs it serves.
A decrease in the rate of nerve impulses results in different symptoms, such as decreased muscle tone and a decreased reflex response, and does not produce inflammation.

The vibrations from a tuning fork placed directly on a vertebra not only may restore the bone's natural resonance, but also may alter the frequency of nerve impulses. This is certainly an area worth researching in the future.

More than a hundred different chiropractic techniques are used for correcting spinal subluxations. Some techniques are characterized as non-force, some are low-force, and others are moderate-force. While some techniques deal with the whole spine, others may be used to correct only the upper cervical spine, and still others may address only the pelvic region. When properly applied, each of these techniques can be of great value.

In my practice, I have found that bone toning with tuning forks not only can be used to correct a subluxation directly, but also can complement hands-on chiropractic adjustments. Bone toning allows the spine to deeply relax and therefore can facilitate adjustments done by hand.

A caveat – if you suspect that a vertebra may be fractured, do not attempt to do any bone toning until you have examined the patient's x-rays. Bone toning should not be used on a fractured bone.

The bone toning that I have been developing involves applying specific frequencies to individual vertebrae. In my studies (and those of other field practitioners of vibrational medicine), tuning forks have proven to be an effective tool for restoring harmonic resonance in the spine. Unfortunately, using tuning forks for extended periods of time is not very practical. What is needed is a device for generating any desired vibrational frequency that then can be focused on a specific location on the body. A hand-held sound generator prototype, based on the personal computer WAV audio device, was developed for me by an electronics engineer. It was programmed to generate the desired frequency at the touch of a button, but the vibrations it produced were found to be too weak to use for bone toning. A second, more powerful device is currently being designed.

To date, my research has focused mostly on identifying the resonant frequencies of the individual vertebrae. The next stage, which I have just begun, is to determine how effective this treatment is for various conditions. Certainly, clinical or controlled trials are needed to determine the best way to apply vibrations for treating subluxations and other dysfunctions of the spine. I hope that other researchers will be stimulated and encouraged to expand this work and determine the most effective means of applying bone toning to other dysfunctions.

Bone Toning Treatments

In my private practice, I have offered bone toning treatments to selected patients. The treatments are relatively quick, lasting from 5 to 15 minutes, and usually are given two to three times a week for several weeks.

Patients have responded to vertebral toning with amazing results. Some reported they were sleeping better than they had for years, some said that their headaches or their pain from temporo-mandibular joint (TMJ) dysfunction had disappeared, and others were happy to find that their neck or back pain had significantly diminished. In order to maintain the beneficial effects of toning, I recommend that the toning be repeated at regular intervals.

Headaches caused by cervical tension are particularly receptive to bone toning. During treatment, the muscles of the neck (particularly the sub-occipital muscles and the trapezius) relax, allowing an increase in nerve and blood flow. Patients often feel quick relief, in some cases after a short period of lightheadedness.

Cases that involve rheumatoid arthritis, lupus, and fibromyalgia also respond well to bone toning treatments. Patients have reported greater muscle relaxation, easier movement of joints, decreased inflammation, and restful sleep. Bone toning also can provide symptomatic relief for conditions such as chronic obstructive pulmonary disease (bronchitis, asthma), heart dysfunctions, renal and reproductive disorders, and abdominal dysfunctions.

In some cases, a dysfunctional heart condition may be due to a weakened impulse from a compressed, stretched, or inflamed spinal nerve exiting from the third or fourth thoracic vertebral segment. Because the nerve is compromised, coherent messages to the heart cannot be received. Bone toning these specific vertebrae may help to establish proper communication between the nervous system and the heart.

One of the most astounding effects of bone toning treatment is the relaxation of the central nervous system and balancing of the autonomic nervous system. For example, one patient who was experiencing tachycardia (fast heartbeat) developed a slower beat and more balanced rhythm. A patient with disorders of the respiratory system who was experiencing difficulty in breathing reported that respiration became easier after a bone toning session. Patients who were suffering from allergies, sinus problems, and headaches also felt relief after one or several treatments. Some patients even claimed that their vision was much clearer.

I feel it would be of great value to perform further research to determine if bone toning can be effective in older patients with degeneration of the spinal bones and discs, bones that may have a significantly diminished resonance response. The need for research with children is just as great. Because children's bones are much more likely to have a vibrant response, bone toning may help young patients with neurological and muscular dysfunctions.

In clinics that perform chiropractic, osteopathic, physical therapy, acupuncture, massage therapy, and bodywork treatments, bone toning can be a valuable way to enhance and augment the success of any standard treatment. No matter what condition is being treated, bone toning can help to restore the body to a more natural, harmonic, and homeostatic state.

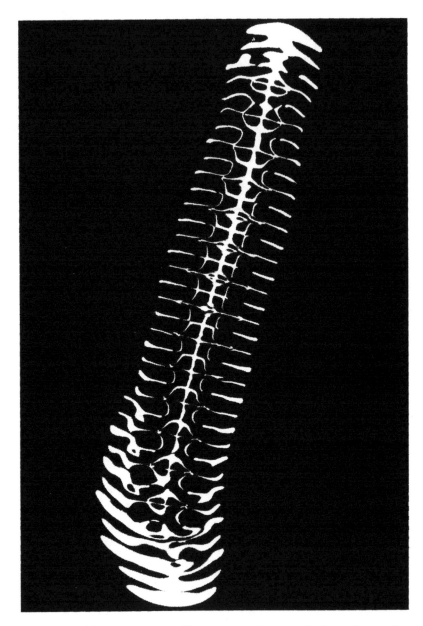

This spine-like image is actually a wave train created when a layer of glycerin is excited by an audible tone. These standing waves, viewed from above, have been illuminated by lighting from the side.

— *From* Cymatics: A Study of Wave Phenomena and Vibrations, by Hans Jenny, © 2001 Macromedia Publishing. Used with permission

CHAPTER 7

MUSCLE TESTING

NO ONE KNOWS WHY or exactly how muscle testing works, but it does. Although the name implies that muscle strength is the primary object of the test, what actually is being tested is the control of muscle function by the nervous system. Muscle testing is used by thousands of chiropractors, physical therapists, homeopathic practitioners, and naturopathic doctors to evaluate specific body functions. When done by a skilled and experienced examiner, muscle testing can identify functional disorders in the nervous and hormonal systems as well as muscular dysfunctions. Muscle testing provides valuable information about which therapy will be most effective to heal the body. It can be used in conjunction with standard medical tests for differential diagnosis and treatment purposes.

A more formal name for muscle testing is "applied kinesiology." The discipline of applied kinesiology is defined by David S. Walther as a system that uses manual muscle testing to evaluate how the body reacts to various stimuli applied to the nervous system. Dr. Walther is the author of a comprehensive textbook, *Applied Kinesiology: Synopsis*.

Another leading researcher in the field, Dr. Walter H. Schmitt Jr., has suggested that applied kinesiology should be defined as functional neurology – the study of how the nervous system controls muscle and body functions. Dr. Schmitt has proposed a conceptual model of the neurophysiological mechanisms that are involved.

The International College of Applied Kinesiology, founded in 1976 to promote the teaching of the discipline and to support clinical and basic research, also defines applied kinesiology as a functional neurological evaluation. More specifically, the College describes its discipline as a diagnostic system using muscle testing as a primary feedback mechanism to determine how a person's body is functioning. The method is concerned mainly with neuromuscular function as it relates to the structural, chemical, and regulatory mechanisms of the nervous system. An applied kinesiology examination requires knowledge of neurology, anatomy, physiology, biochemistry, and biomechanics, and it is performed in conjunction with standard medical examination procedures such as x-rays and lab tests.

The original muscle testing techniques were developed to evaluate muscle strength in polio patients. A paper describing a method of testing muscular strength in infantile paralysis patients was published in 1915 in the *Journal of the American Medical Association*, and improved methods for determining precise muscle strength continued to be published in medical journals for the next 40 years. In 1949, two physical therapists, H.O. Kendall and F.M.P. Kendall, published an excellent book, *Muscles – Testing and Function*, which became the basis for modern muscle testing techniques.

George J. Goodheart Jr., a chiropractor in Detroit, began using the Kendall technique to evaluate muscle strength in his patients. He astutely surmised that the muscle test might "predict" whether a particular muscle group was functioning properly. Further testing revealed that muscle testing can be used to uncover other dysfunctions. Goodheart refined the technique and called it "applied kinesiology." After presenting his findings at the charter meeting of the American Chiropractic Association in 1964, he began giving workshops to teach others how to use this technique in their healing work.

In addition to giving lectures and workshops, Goodheart continued to conduct original research, developing tests and treatments for many functional disorders. He extensively studied the relationship between muscle response, the acupuncture meridians, and the health of the vital systems (immune, nervous, cardiovascular, and cerebrospinal fluid). He also found that muscle testing can be used to evaluate the body's nutritional state. In the mid-1980s he proposed a holographic theory for how the brain maintains awareness of all aspects of the body, and he described how such a holographic model of the nervous system can explain why muscle testing works as a diagnostic tool.

One of the standard muscle testing techniques is the arm-extension method, although individual muscles or muscle groups in other parts of the body – legs, back, neck, fingers, or feet, for example – also can be used. With the arm-extension method, a patient, who may be standing, sitting, or lying down, is asked to extend an arm. The practitioner puts his hand on top of the extended arm and asks the patient to resist having the arm forced down. The arm should be kept strong and extended straight out. When the practitioner applies even and firm pressure, the patient usually will lock the muscles of the arm and easily resist the applied pressure. When this happens, the muscle test is said to be "strong." If the arm collapses when pressure is applied, another limb should be used for the muscle testing, and the reason for the "weak" response should be investigated later.

The practitioner initially applies pressure several times to determine the strength and tone of the muscle group. This is done by increasing the pressure when resistance is felt. The rate at which the pressure is increased is critical. The initial increase must be slow enough to allow the patient's nervous system to lock the muscle against the pressure, and the subsequent increase in pressure should be at a rate that gives the muscle enough time to adapt. A quick increase in pressure after locking has occurred will overcome the muscle before it can adapt to the changing pressure, whereas a slower increase in pressure will allow it to adapt as much as it can and produce a true "strong" or "weak" response.

Muscle testing is both a science and art. To be successful, the practitioner must develop a set of skills in the timing and application of the testing force. Sometimes the response from the client's muscle can be subtle, and a good practitioner is able to detect this. A "strong" response in muscle testing consists of what is called a "lock-in" phase. A "weak" response is when the arm or muscle tested loses strength when pressure is applied. This can result in either a dropping of the arm or up-and-down oscillation of the arm.

It is important for the practitioner to stay neutral when performing a muscle test in order to get clear results. Through the course of hundreds of tests, I have found that merely thinking a negative thought will produce a "weak" muscle test, while a positive thought will produce a "strong" response.

After the practitioner has determined the tone and strength of a muscle that tests "strong," it can be used as an indicator to test for dysfunctions and imbalances in the body. The patient is asked to touch a particular part of the body, and the muscle test is repeated. For instance, if the patient touches the skin over the thyroid gland and the muscle test response is "weak," that indicates a dysfunction in the thyroid. A person with a gastric ulcer will have a "weak" muscle response when he touches the skin over the stomach. This technique, called therapy localization, generally works well over pathological areas.

A variety of muscle testing techniques may be used. One alternative that a person can use to test herself or himself is called the finger "O" test. The tips of the thumb and the small finger of one hand are pressed together to form a circle, and the thumb and forefinger of the other hand are inserted into the circle with the tips pressed together to form a second, locked-in circle. The person now mentally asks a question that has a yes or no answer and steadily pulls the hands apart. If the fingers break apart, then the answer is no. If they remain locked, the answer is yes.

In muscle testing, a response is rarely only slightly strong or slightly weak, but at times the response may be jerky, with a progressive weakness. This is an indication that the person being tested is calling up all his or her strength to overcome the spontaneous weakness. This jerky response is very different from the normal "strong" response based on a locked muscle. Certain conditions, however, such as dehydration or the presence of drugs, can make a person's responses to manual muscle testing erratic. It is important not to use a muscle that is dysfunctional, because the response is likely to be compromised and the testing may cause further injury.

A number of researchers have attempted to quantify applied kinesiology using devices to apply the force or pressure. These studies have not been successful, in part because the devices do not apply the pressure incrementally and thus do not allow the muscles to adapt to the changing force.

I also propose that one way to objectify muscle testing is to use a mechanical device designed so that it can apply a variety of specific pressures or a steadily increasing pressure. The use of graduated pressures could help to determine whether muscle testing is subjective. Another approach for quantifying muscle testing would be to develop a hand-held device that continuously measures the pressure that a practitioner applies.

The International College of Applied Kinesiology has supported research using electromyography, or EMG, to measure muscle responses during manual muscle testing. One of their findings is that the "weak" muscle response is fundamentally different from a fatigued muscle response. Further research using direct physiological measurements such as EMG and skin conductance are warranted. Other researchers have used a computerized dynamometer or similar instruments to assess the reliability of manual muscle testing.

Muscle testing often is used to determine what vitamins, herbs, supplements, and other nutrients are needed by, or depleted in, the subject. The muscle response is "strong" to substances that a person's body recognizes as being therapeutic. On the other hand, harmful substances produce an instant "weak" test response. For example, when a person touches a potential allergen and shows a "weak" muscle test, that indicates that the person is allergic to that substance. This procedure will work even when the practitioner or the person being tested does not know what the substance is.

Occasionally, a muscle will test "weak" because of systemic imbalances. I have found great value in using a muscle that tests "weak" (and is not dysfunctional), because this gives me even greater confidence when a nutrient, for example, produces a "strong" test.

In the 1970s, Dr. John Diamond, a psychiatrist, began using muscle testing for diagnosing his patients. He conducted experiments on how a variety of psychological or mental stimuli – such as music, facial expressions, art, tone of voice, and emotional stress – affected the muscle test response. He discovered that positive, or healthy, emotional stimuli produce a "strong" test response and negative stimuli a "weak" response. His results led him to create a new discipline that he named "behavioral kinesiology."

Dr. Diamond found that certain designs or symbols – a pitchfork, say – would produce a "weak" muscle test response in every person he tested, while other designs – a cross, for instance – would always produce a "strong" response. He also noted that subjects hearing a speaker telling the truth tested "strong," whereas they tested "weak" when they listened to a speaker who told lies.

These muscle test responses to truth and falsehood caught the interest of another psychiatrist, Dr. David R. Hawkins, a therapist and lecturer who in 1973 co-authored the book *Orthomolecular Psychiatry* with the Nobel prize winner Linus Pauling. Dr. Hawkins saw in muscle testing the potential to bridge the physical body and the mind, viewing it as a tool to map levels of human consciousness. He found that the true/false response to statements is accurate even when the person being tested has no knowledge of the topic and that the test response is independent of the person's opinions on the topic. Dr. Hawkins feels that for the first time there is a tool for distinguishing between truth and falsity in an objective way and across cultures. His investigations are based on the use of muscle testing to determine the truth or falsity of a declarative statement to which the answer must be a clear yes or no. A question in any other form produces unreliable results. His refinements of the procedure allow calibration of the relative truth or energy of statements, ideologies, beliefs, attitudes, feelings, relationships, and other situations.

Dr. Hawkins undertook a large-scale investigation to calibrate levels of human consciousness. The result is a logarithmic scale from 1 to 1000 to measure levels of human awareness. In his book *Power vs. Force, The Hidden Determinants of Human Behavior*, he states: "The notion that our actions are based on thoughtful decisions is a grand illusion. The mind acts much more rapidly than that." Making rapid choices on the basis of millions of bits of data is far beyond the capacity of conscious comprehension. "The decision-making process is a function of consciousness itself," Hawkins writes. Moment-to-moment decision-making is dominated by energy patterns, or attractor fields, within consciousness itself. "These patterns," he continues, "can be identified, described, and calibrated; out of that information arises a totally new understanding of human behavior, history, and the destiny of mankind."

According to Dr. Hawkins, the validity of muscle testing is well established. It is repeatable and universal. He reports that the reliability of the testing experience never ceases to amaze the observer. "The response has proven cross-culturally valid in any population and consistent over time," he writes.

One of the astounding things about muscle testing is the immediacy and consistency of the results. This has been confirmed by a number of double-blind studies in which experienced practitioners performed muscle tests on the same group of subjects. In most of these studies, there was an 80 percent or better agreement in the test results.

Muscle testing has gained widespread acceptance among professionals in various specialties because of its simplicity, reproducibility, cost effectiveness, and uncanny ability to detect dysfunction within our energetic, emotional, and physical bodies. Unfortunately, this easy-to-use diagnostic tool has not gained much acceptance in mainstream medicine. Perhaps the lack of a physiological model for explaining how muscle testing works is responsible for the lack of interest by the medical profession. It is worth noting, however, that doctors in mainstream medicine treat pain on a daily basis, and yet they have no convincing explanatory model for diagnosing pain or predicting its severity. Instead, they have to rely on the subjective reports of patients.

The body is capable of recognizing the subtle energy fields with which it can resonate. The spine is the central axis of the physical body and is intimately connected to the nervous system. The muscular system is used as an indicator of this resonance. During muscle testing, what actually is being tested is the central nervous system, along with the resonant frequencies on a cellular level. Regardless of the subject's or practitioner's awareness or the intention of either, it is the body and its innate wisdom that responds. In muscle testing, clearly it is not a meeting of our minds. What I find of great value in muscle testing is that it takes the ego out of the practitioner. I am not telling patients what works for them, their bodies are telling me.

Muscle testing is a handy tool at our fingertips. I am astounded and continuously amazed that we are able to assess through muscle testing an infinite amount of information by deeply listening, tapping into our innate intelligence. Through muscle testing, I gain valuable information about each patient's present condition, which allows me to diagnose accurately and to treat the patient more effectively. Often the diagnosis is later confirmed by x-rays or laboratory tests. When properly applied, muscle testing provides immediate and useful information about each patient's diagnosis and treatment.

Muscle testing has proved to me to be an accurate, non-subjective test for accessing information that resides in our conscious and unconscious thoughts. In a way, muscle testing serves as my polygraph, my lie detector. The polygraph instrument measures visceral reactions, such as pulse rate, sweating, and breath. Nevertheless, the results of this instrument's tests often are inaccurate or misleading because of the variability of the "stress response" of the individual being tested. In addition, you can cheat in a lie detection session by gently moving the toes of one foot every time you answer a question truthfully and not moving the toes when you lie – which will confuse the baseline used to evaluate lies.

In our courts, witnesses are asked to place a hand on the Bible and swear to tell the truth and nothing but the truth. There is no way of telling whether this improves the chances of truth telling, especially when the witness is an agnostic or an atheist. I think it would be worthwhile to use muscle testing as an alternative. The witness would be instructed to hold out an arm, then would be asked, *Do you swear to tell the truth, the whole truth, and nothing but the truth?* If the arm remains "strong," truth telling can be expected. If the arm tests "weak," beware!

CHAPTER 8

PROCEDURES, CASE HISTORIES, AND RESEARCH

WHEN A PATIENT ENTERS MY OFFICE, it is essential for me to perform a thorough examination. After I have reviewed the patient's medical history, I make my evaluation through careful observation, very attentive listening (this is where you will receive the most valuable information about the patient), and palpation (static and motion). I also employ appropriate orthopedic and neurological tests, including x-rays. After problem areas have been identified, I decide on the most appropriate therapeutic measures.

When bone toning is indicated, the procedure is carefully explained to the patient. I use muscle testing along with palpation, x-rays, or an electronic device such as a Nervo-scope to confirm the location of any subluxation.

When I am looking for a subluxated vertebra or for a vertebra with loss of tone, I simultaneously muscle-test as I touch the vertebra. With the patient sitting up, I usually use an arm for muscle-testing the cervical vertebrae. Next I have the patient lie face down while I test the lumbar region, usually using a leg for muscle testing. To test the vertebrae of the thoracic spine, I use the arm test for the upper part and the leg muscle test for the middle to lower parts. In some cases, I find it useful to have an assistant touch the vertebrae while I perform muscle testing. When the muscle test response is "strong," it is very likely that there is no subluxation at that location. When the muscle test gives a "weak" response, that means a dysfunctional vertebra has been found.

Bone toning can be performed with the patient sitting up or lying down. The appropriate tuning fork is tapped and applied to the subluxated vertebra. If the patient has a headache, for instance, treatment of the upper cervical spine – the C1, C2 vertebrae – is most often indicated, or in some cases the thoracic vertebrae may need treatment. Often a single application of the tuning fork for about 10 seconds is enough to produce the desired results. When there is some kind of resistance that might dampen the effect of the acoustic vibrations, such as a thick layer of fat or muscle tension over the treatment area, the tuning fork may have to be applied several times, each application lasting between 10 and 30 seconds. It may be necessary to strike the tuning fork several times rapidly to attain a strong, sustained vibration.

As I tone the bone with the tuning fork, I continue to perform muscle testing. The muscle response will continue to be strong until the vertebra has completely absorbed the vibration needed to support it. When a vertebra has been completely toned, the muscle test will suddenly show a weakened response, meaning that the body has recognized when the stimulation of vibrations has reached its optimal effect and no further toning is necessary. When the optimal effect has been reached, over-stimulation of the vertebra produces the weakened muscle response.

When the bone toning has been completed, I muscle-test again to determine if the treatment has been effective. I touch the appropriate vibrating fork against the treated vertebra and muscle-test simultaneously. If the test response is weak, that indicates that the vibrations have had the optimal effect and the additional vibration in the test is causing over-stimulation. However, if the muscle test is strong, that indicates that the vertebra needs additional treatment. In addition to muscle testing, the effects of bone toning can be evaluated by palpation, x-rays, or an electronic device that is designed to detect subluxations.

There are three essential elements in every bone toning session, as is the case for any treatment using vibrational medicine: the frequency used, the intent of the practitioner, and the receptivity of the client.

Selecting the correct frequency for a particular vertebra is of utmost importance. Using an inappropriate frequency will have, at best, little or no effect, and it could even produce a harmful effect. Another important aspect of the treatment is the amount of stimulation that is applied. Too little is likely to be ineffective, whereas too much could cause over-stimulation. The correct amount of stimulation is determined empirically. With experience, a practitioner of bone toning will be able to quickly ascertain how much vibration to apply.

The practitioner's primary intention must be the patient's health and well-being. Such intention brings clarity to the practitioner, who then focuses on the patient's vital interests without ego and without judgment. As a practitioner who is part of the healing equation, I have found that it is essential to be able to step aside, to get "mind" out of the way, and allow an innate healing and intelligence to guide me.

The patient's receptivity plays a vital role in this type of treatment, as it does in any healing process. The patient must be open and willing to receive the therapy. That does not mean that vibrational medicine is "faith healing." I consider chiropractic medicine to be vibrational medicine because a specific speed, along with force, is needed in order to give a correction or adjustment to a particular vertebra, thus relieving pressure on the nervous system and allowing the body to naturally heal itself. I have even seen the benefits of adjustments to horses, dogs, and cats – without their belief in chiropractic!

Vibrational medicine produces beneficial results even when a patient has initial doubts. With bone toning, the results are sometimes immediate, but in other cases repeated treatments are needed. In a few cases, the bone toning appears to have no effect. Nevertheless, 9 out of 10 patients in my practice report an improved feeling of well-being after a bone toning treatment.

I offer bone toning with tuning forks to patients who I think may benefit from it. The choice is the patient's, of course. Many people who have heard about bone toning from friends or relatives come to my office for the treatment. I also receive phone calls and e-mails from people who have learned about bone toning from my websites (www.drwieder.com and www.bone-toning.com).

Here are six case histories that are representative of patients who received bone toning in my office.

CASE 1: A young woman who was diagnosed with multiple sclerosis came to me with a complaint of numbness in both hands. I gave her a thorough evaluation using orthopedic and neurological tests, which revealed fixations and subluxations in her cervical and thoracic spine at the level of C1 and T1. I treated these two vertebrae with the appropriate (130.81 Hz) tuning fork for approximately 10 seconds. In only a few moments, the subject said that complete sensation had returned to both of her hands. The effect of this single treatment lasted for several months, but the numbness returned after she took antibiotics prescribed by her physician. After the numbness continued for a few days, she came to my office once again for a bone toning treatment. I repeated the same protocol, and both hands regained full sensation.

CASE 2: A middle-aged woman complained of headaches, decreased motion in her neck, and inability to sleep through the night. A thorough examination, including x-rays, revealed that the patient's head was tilted to the left, with right rotation. When I applied compression her cervical spine (neck), she reported significant pain. Her x-rays revealed slight degeneration in the lower cervical spine, with malpositioned first and second cervical vertebrae. Touch examination of the spine identified a fixation of the second cervical vertebra. I applied the appropriate tuning forks to the first cervical vertebra (130.81 Hz) and the second cervical vertebra (146.83 Hz). Within seconds the headache ceased, and the patient's head was aligned – with no rotation and no head tilt. When I again applied compression the cervical spine, the patient said she felt very little pain. On a subsequent visit to my office, the woman reported having slept better than she had for years.

CASE 3: A 45-year-old, exceptionally tall and thin gentleman had moderate to severe lower back pain for several months. He said that walking, standing, or sitting for long periods increased the pain, as did transitional positions such as sitting-to-stand or lying-to-sit. The pain eased when he was still. When I touched and motioned his spine, I noted that there was decreased motion of the sacroiliac joints. The last lumbar vertebra (L5) was fixated to the right, and the range of motion of the lumbar spine was decreased by about 20 degrees to the left. Some inflammation was apparent. The patient's x-rays and MRI were negative for soft tissue, disc, or bone pathology. I applied the appropriate (233.08 Hz) tuning fork to the spinous process of the L5 vertebra for approximately 10 seconds, then repeated the procedure two more times. The patient reported an immediate relaxation of the lower back muscles. When I motioned his spine again, the vertebra and sacroiliac joints moved freely, and the swelling was no longer present.

CASE 4: A young woman said that she had difficulty sleeping, a lack of energy, and severe pain and soreness in her muscles. She had been diagnosed by her physician as having a condition known as fibromyalgia, which can present itself as mild or debilitating. This sensitive patient had many exquisitely tender points when I palpated several different areas. Generalized edema was present in the soft tissues. I treated her several times per week using tuning forks with the frequency of 196 Hz for the fifth cervical and fifth thoracic vertebrae, and 233.08 Hz for the fifth lumbar vertebra. The first week, the patient reported deep sleep and a good night's rest. She said she felt more energized, but her muscle soreness remained. By the end of the second week, she was able to work in her home and office without much soreness in her muscles. After the third week, her joints moved more freely and her muscle soreness was much reduced. She stated that she had not felt this well for years.

CASE 5: An overweight, elderly woman was suffering from dizziness, headaches, and tinnitus (perception of high-pitched buzzing sounds, for which there is no standard treatment). The intensity of the perceived sound in tinnitus can be so severe that some people attempt suicide. When I took the patient's vital signs, I found that her blood pressure and pulse rate were slightly elevated. She said that she was taking a variety of medications, including aspirin. Her diet was not particularly nutritional. She smoked a pack of cigarettes a day and drank about six cups of coffee. All of these factors may trigger tinnitus, although none are known to be the cause. When I examined her spine, I found that the first cervical vertebra was significantly rotated in relation to her second cervical vertebra. I applied the appropriate (130.81 Hz) tuning fork to the C1 vertebra, with dramatic results. With just one treatment, her dizziness was greatly reduced, the headache disappeared, and the tinnitus was reduced.

CASE STUDY 6: An overweight, middle-aged male had lower back pain as well as numbness and tingling sensations in both hands and feet. He also had a history of diabetes mellitus type II, and he restricted his diet at times to control the disease. My examination revealed that his deep tendon reflexes were slightly diminished in both the upper and lower extremities, and his muscle strength was weak in the legs. X-rays showed mild to moderate degeneration of the lumbar (lower) spine. I recommended that we try bone-toning three times a week for several months. The treatment consisted of applying frequencies of 185.00 Hz and 207.65 Hz to the third and fourth lumbar vertebrae. After three months of treatment, the patient reported feeling increased sensation in his hands and feet and a significant decrease in his lower back pain. Although his deep tendon reflexes remained diminished, the patient regained strength and tone in his leg muscles, especially his quadriceps and calf muscles. In an exploratory research study that I conducted with my colleague, Mark R. Filippi, DC, I used two measuring devices and a self-rated wellness questionnaire as well as muscle testing to determine the effects of bone toning. The primary device was the PulStar Force Recording and Analysis System, or PulStarFRAS, invented by Joseph Evans, a bioengineer. The device delivers a low-force impulse to measure the tension of muscles along the spine. It also can be used to deliver a continuous train of impulses to adjust vertebrae. PulStarFRAS is manufactured and sold by a company called Sense Technology (www.pulstarfras.com). In the analysis mode, the PulStar generates a graphical display of the relative compliance of each vertebra tested.

The second device used in the study was the Insight 7000 Subluxation Station, which measures surface EMGs (muscle response) along the spine and also heat differences along the spine using infrared thermography. The wellness self-rating employed in the study was made using one of the Rand Health Surveys.

Dr. Filippi and I tracked a group of nine volunteers over a three-month period, seeing each a total of 12 times. During the initial session, each person was evaluated by the PulStarFRAS instrument and Insight 7000 Subluxation Station to establish a baseline, and each also completed the wellness self-rating survey.

Each of the nine volunteers received bone toning using tuning forks during each session, except for two subjects who received a PulStar adjustment for two sessions. The subjects wore medical gowns to allow for skin contact. Muscle testing was performed each time a tuning fork was placed on a vertebra. Subjects were also pre- and post-tested with the PulStar at each session. Insight 7000 measurements were made at only four of the 12 sessions.

Overall, the Insight EMG and thermography data showed that bone toning with tuning forks decreased muscle tension along the spine. The data from the wellness surveys were inconclusive. The

PulStarFRAS results, however, were dramatic – in most of the subjects, bone toning altered vertebral compliance. The post-toning graphs showed relaxation of muscles that were tense and stiff in the pre-test graphs. Also, muscles that had been slack showed increased tone in the post-toning graphs.

The PulStar data suggest that the vibrations of the tuning forks are capable of bringing harmony to the spinal muscles. Further studies certainly are warranted. The PulStar device can be used not only to measure the effect of bone toning, but also as a means to obtain objective data that may validate the results of muscle testing.

Other devices may also be useful for measuring the effect of bone toning or for complementing muscle testing. The Nervo-scope, which measures the difference in heat on either side of the spine, is one such device.

Not all the treatments received by my clients have produced dramatic or even very good results. But more than 90 percent of my patients report a remembrance of parts of themselves that have long been forgotten, and they experience a more integrated sense of wholeness.

CHAPTER 9

VIBRATION IN CONVENTIONAL MEDICINE

CURRENT RESEARCH IN THE FIELDS OF PHYSICS and biology is confirming that the animate world comprises dynamic and sometimes complex energy systems. The human body is composed of subatomic, atomic, and molecular particles, all of which vibrate and oscillate at their own frequencies. Because each person is unique, all of us have our own distinct energy patterns.

In vibrational medicine, the human body is perceived as an unfolding and dynamic resonant system. When the components of the body are in harmony, there is an internal balance, or homeostasis, that produces a stable and vital state of health. When the parts of the body/mind/spirit are not in harmony, we experience dis-ease.

Homeostasis is a fundamental concept in modern biology, but the idea that inner harmony or balance is necessary to maintain health goes back to prehistoric times. The scientific version of the idea had its beginning in the 19th century, when the French physiologist Claude Bernard observed that the body fluids were of a constant composition. Bernard believed that this constancy was essential to living organisms. In the early 20th century, Walter B. Cannon, an American physiologist, coined the term *homeostasis* to describe self-regulating systems in living organisms. Cannon believed that the body tries to maintain an equilibrium, or balance, in all its systems.

Homeostasis operates at all levels within the living organism, from the molecular to the systemic. It regulates the concentrations of nutrients, gases, hormones, and other substances in the body fluids. The immune system and the nervous system continuously rely on homeostatic mechanisms. When an imbalance occurs, the body seeks to return to the original homeostatic conditions.

The various techniques used in vibrational medicine are designed to help the body return to its harmonious, homeostatic, healthy state. Chanting or toning, for example, produces a strong internal vibration that affects every cell and helps restore the natural harmony of the body, mind, and spirit.

Bone serves as the structure that provides support and stability, as the place where our blood cells are made, and as a storehouse for calcium and phosphorus. Bone also is a superb conductor of vibrations. Bones allow our bodies to be vehicles in which sound can penetrate to the deepest spaces within us, making changes on a cellular level and possibly regenerating our neural pathways.

In the skull, the sinus cavities create rich resonances that greatly enhance and strengthen the sounds generated by the vocal cords. The bones of the spine conduct vibrations up and down the length of the body. This flow of vibrations is disrupted when a subluxation of the spine exists. Correcting the subluxation allows the natural vibrational pattern to be restored; thus, the healing process can be accelerated by applying the correct vibrational frequency to the subluxated vertebrae. Often the subluxation can be corrected by simply applying a vibrating tuning fork to the "out of tune" vertebra.

Orthopedic surgeons have recently begun using oscillating electromagnetic fields to accelerate the healing of fractured bones. This is a beautiful and concrete example of how energetic vibrational messages carry information to specific tissues. In order for healing to occur, the electromagnetic vibrations of the "bone stimulators" must be set at a precise frequency. If the frequency is set incorrectly, the bone will weaken instead of heal.

The use of electromagnetic energy to stimulate the healing of broken bones was pioneered by Dr. Robert Becker, an orthopedic surgeon who was deeply interested in the effects of various kinds of energy fields on the human body. His most significant discovery was that the body has a direct-current electrical control system. He demonstrated that a person under anesthesia had markedly different direct-current potentials around the head. Even hypnotically anesthetized persons had changed electrical potentials. Becker reasoned that because hypnosis is an altered state of consciousness, there may be a correlation between states of consciousness and changes in the body's direct-current potentials. He concluded that a direct-current system may be an alternative pathway for sending messages between the brain and any damaged bone or tissue. A carrier of the direct-current messages may be the glial cells. Becker found that the slow voltage changes observed in glial nerve cells (which support nerves) can be modified by applying a magnetic field, and he later demonstrated complete anesthesia in animals using only applied magnetic fields.

Several different kinds of vibrations are used in medical diagnosis and treatment. These vibrational ranges can be categorized as sound, ultrasound, and electromagnetic (including heat, light, and x-rays). The vibrations we call sound are low in frequency, from 20 to 20,000 Hz (cycles per second).

Ultrasound, or ultrasonic, waves are vibrations above 20,000 Hz. This frequency is outside the normal human hearing range, although some mammals, such as whales, can hear ultrasound frequencies up to about 50,000 Hz. Medical ultrasound devices can generate frequencies up to 20 Megahertz (20 million cycles per second).

Ultrasound is best known for its use in obstetrics and for diagnosis of tumors. Ultrasound pictures of the fetus are taken almost routinely to monitor prenatal development, particularly if there is reason for concern about abnormalities.

Ultrasound is used therapeutically to apply mechanical effects that generate heat in deep tissues. It is routinely used by physical therapists to reduce pain and swelling and to accelerate the healing of wounds.

Cataracts are a major cause of blindness in older people. Today, cataracts are removed surgically using ultrasound. In a procedure called phacoemulsification, the eye surgeon makes a tiny incision near the lens of the eye and inserts a tiny ultrasonic probe. The ultrasonic vibrations break up the lens and the cataract, and the debris is sucked out by the probe. The surgeon then inserts a plastic lens that is customized to give the patient normal vision.

Ultrasound also is used to break up kidney stones without invasive surgery. In this procedure, called lithotripsy, high-energy ultrasonic waves are directed at the kidney. Stones that have formed there absorb these waves and shatter into pieces that usually are small enough to pass through the urethra during normal urination. The presence of different kinds of tissue in the body, however, makes it difficult to precisely focus a high-energy ultrasound pulse. A new approach uses a technique called time-reversed acoustics, which records the echo of a sound wave and reverses it before transmitting it back to where it originated. Because the returning ultrasound pulse is a mirror image of the echo, the tissues that had bent and distorted the echo will now guide the time-reversed pulse back to the location from which the echo originated.

In this procedure, which is also used to treat gallstones, the ultrasonic device first sends a low-energy pulse and then records the reflection from the kidney stone. The device then amplifies the pulse and reflects it back to the exact location that caused the reflection. The high-energy, time-reversed ultrasound pulse is automatically focused by the intervening tissues, causing the kidney stone to resonate and shatter. The device then repeats the process until all the stones have been destroyed.

Time-reversed ultrasound is also being used to identify and treat tumors in the heart or other tissues that are not functioning properly. The time-reversed pulse is capable of heating and destroying the malfunctioning tissue without causing damage to the surrounding heart cells. Research is now being conducted on the use of time-reversed ultrasound to destroy brain tumors, but special techniques are still needed to overcome the distortion of sound waves created by the skull.

It may be possible to develop similar methods for treating the spine. Various frequencies of sound or ultrasound can be pulsed to the spine, and the echoes captured and analyzed. It may be possible to target an individual vertebra with a specific frequency using a time-reversed signal. Perhaps we may discover that amplified time-reversed sounds can be effective for treating conditions such as osteoporosis and degenerative joint disease.

Ultrasound also can be used to kill bacteria and other pathogens that are in a good sound-conducting medium, such as water. Researchers have developed a technique that destroys the spores of harmful bacteria such as anthrax when they are compressed between paper or cloth fibers. It is likely that ultrasound can be used to kill other pathogens. Further research is needed to identify the frequencies that cause various pathogens to self-destruct.

Light is another form of vibrational energy. Compared to sound and ultrasound, light vibrates at very high frequencies – millions of times higher, in fact. Today, lasers are increasingly being used for surgical and other medical treatments. Lasers emit a special type of light called coherent light, in which the waves move in step with one another, like soldiers marching in step. Lasers also can emit a single frequency of light, something that is very hard to achieve using other light sources. Laser light can be focused to a very small diameter, and its immense power can vaporize the object it is focused on. Ophthalmologists use lasers for surgical treatment of glaucoma and detached retinas, or to improve a person's eyesight by correcting imperfections in the cornea. Surgeons also use laser scalpels to remove organs, such as gall bladders, that have become diseased.

Within the medical profession, the use of vibrational tools is still rather limited. Generally, powerful vibrations are used to image body parts or to destroy diseased parts. Some members of the medical profession, however, have begun to recognize the potential of using non-invasive, natural therapies. Oliver Sacks, a leading neurologist, has testified at a U.S. Senate committee about the healing power of music in treating neurological disorders such as Parkinson's disease. He described one woman whose EEG readings usually were flat, almost comatose-like, but who would revert to a normal EEG pattern when she imagined she was playing music. Most of the day she sat motionless, but when she was seated at a piano, she would play beautifully for hours.

Dr. Sacks became aware of the potential healing power of music from his own experience. While hiking (actually, running away from a bull) he broke a leg that healed badly, and his mind refused to recognize that the dysfunctional leg was part of his body. Sacks spent many months consulting other physicians, most of whom simply ignored his problem. One day Sacks noted that his leg moved when he was listening to classical music, and he used that discovery to regain the use of his leg.

Another example of the power of low-energy vibrations comes from researchers at Harvard Medical School. Working with a vibrating pad from Afferent Corp., they demonstrated that vibrations applied to the soles of the foot improve a person's ability to maintain balance. The vibrations were subthreshold, meaning they were almost imperceptible. Both young and elderly subjects exhibited better balance, but the effect was notably greater among the elderly. The team's findings, published in the British medical journal

The Lancet, indicate that vibrating shoe insoles may be beneficial for people whose sense of balance has begun to deteriorate. It is my hope that in the future, research will validate that each vertebra does indeed respond to a specific vibrational frequency, and that this knowledge will help to treat patients non-invasively and help restore harmony to the backbone of humanity.

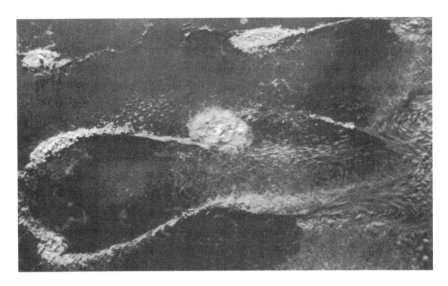

Vibrations generated by crystal oscillators that propagate continuous waves create currents of flowing sand, which form rotational patterns that resemble spiral galaxies.

— *From* Cymatics: A Study of Wave Phenomena and Vibrations, *by Hans Jenny, © 2001 Macromedia Publishing. Used with permission.*

CHAPTER 10

NEUROBIOLOGY OF VIBRATIONAL HEALING

We Chiropractors work with the subtle substance of the soul. We release the imprisoned impulse – the tiny rivulet of force – that emanates from the mind and flows over the nerves to cells and stirs them into life. We deal with the majestic power that transforms common food into living, loving clay; that robes the Earth with beauty, and hues and scents the flowers with the glory of the air.

In the dim, dark, distant long ago when the sun first bowed to the morning star, this power spoke and there was life; it quickened the slime of the sea and dust of the Earth and drove the cell to union with its fellows in countless living forms. Through eons of time, it finned the fish and winged the bird and fanged the beast. Endlessly it worked, evolving its forms until it produced the crowing glory of them all. With tireless energy it blows the bubble of each individual life and then silently, relentlessly dissolves the form, and absorbs the spirit into itself again....

"The Truth," poetically stated by B. J. Palmer,
son of the founder of Chiropractic

WHEN THE HUMAN BODY is viewed as a dynamic and unfolding resonant system of vibrations, one can compare it to an orchestrated symphony. Every cell, every molecule, every tissue, every bone dances with a specific frequency and will produce a certain "tone" when stimulated. Thus, vibrational medicine works at a deep, cellular level where molecular properties are being changed by vibrations. Keep in mind that it is not just our bodies that are affected by vibration, but also our minds, spirits, and etheric fields.

In physics, vibrations are a fundamental property of energy and matter. Light is made up of photons that vibrate at very high frequencies. What we call heat is nothing more than the vibration of atoms and molecules. Even subatomic particles such as bosons and quarks and all the other elementary building blocks of matter vibrate.

Vibration in the form of sound waves played a role in the creation of the universe as we know it. Recent satellite images of the far edge of the universe show that temperature variations shortly after the Big Bang were created by sound waves in the primordial plasma, and these temperature variations led to the creation of the first stars and galaxies.

Even more striking is the discovery of sound waves being emitted by a supermassive black hole in the center of the Perseus cluster. An x-ray image taken by NASA shows a regular pattern of pressure, or acoustic, waves in the hot gas surrounding the black hole. The sound waves are created not by the black hole itself but by the spiraling hot gases on the periphery. The frequency of the sound waves is one pulse every 10 million years (a sound only God can hear!), and this turns out to be a constant B-flat with a loudness similar to that of human speech. Where regularity in the acoustic pressure waves exists, there is a corresponding musical tone. The sound waves die out rapidly, however, and their pitch is far, far below human hearing – 57 octaves below the middle-C on a piano. Even though we cannot hear it, the sound emitted by the Perseus cluster is the deepest note yet found in the universe.

Astrophysicists expect to find other black holes that are generating sound waves. In the meantime, scientists Phil Uttley and Ian McHardy are trying to gain an understanding of x-ray emissions from black holes by transcribing the emissions into musical notes, with a higher pitch representing a higher x-ray output. The pattern of notes has a musical quality, they say. Changes in notes and pitch are similar to those in most kinds of music. The note equivalents of x-ray emissions from small stellar black holes vary on a time scale of seconds, whereas those from supermassive black holes vary on a scale of millions of seconds. Another kind of music has been detected in the magnetic fields of our solar system. Astronomers call it flicker noise, and some call it a kind of background music.

Acoustic waves ripple in all directions for thousands of miles across the surface of our sun when violent solar flares erupt. Even the Earth hums a tune. Sound waves inside the Earth have been detected with seismographs, but scientists are unsure how they are created. Some have proposed that sound waves in the atmosphere are transmitted into the Earth, while others say that the pounding of ocean waves may be the source. The subsurface sound waves emit a very low frequency, about one-hundredth of a Hertz – far below the human threshold of hearing.

On Earth, the movement of atoms and molecules orchestrates life. There are special molecules that play the role of messenger in our bodies. The vital organs release into the bloodstream a variety of hormones that regulate our body functions. The immune system releases antibodies and other molecules that detect and attack pathogens, and the nervous system releases molecules that trigger electrochemical impulses in nerve cells. Many parts of the body produce tiny molecules called cytokines that serve as messengers to other parts of the body and to the brain.

But chemical and electrical messages are not the only means of communication found in our body. There also are resonant systems that act on the body as a whole. The 12 meridians of Chinese acupuncture are energetic pathways throughout the body that connect to the vital organs and link specific body functions. The meridians allow an acupuncturist to treat vital organs from parts of the body that are distant from the organs being treated. Another communication system within the body is based on sympathetic vibrations. The beating of the heart, the ebb and flow of

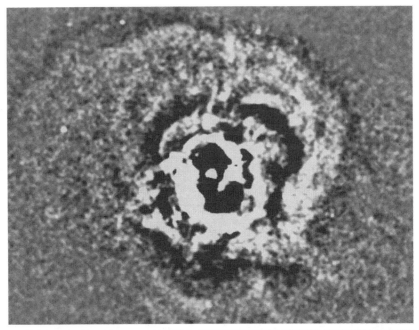

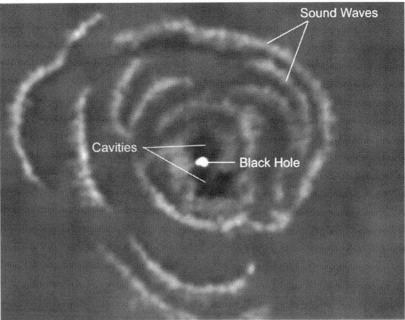

Spiraling gases near a supermassive black hole in the center of the Perseus cluster (top) generate sound waves that are a constant B-flat, but 57 octaves lower than middle-C. Artist's rendering (bottom) delineates the sound waves (NASA images).

cerebrospinal fluid, and the expansion and contraction of the diaphragm all produce mechanical, acoustic waves – vibrations that flow throughout the body.

Many therapists make use of resonance and vibratory energy, whether their treatments are based on touch, aroma, heat, light, or sound, as James L. Oschman states eloquently in his illuminating book *Energy Medicine, The Scientific Basis*:

> A massage therapist touches and rubs the tissue, a herbalist applies an extract of a plant, an acupuncturist applies a needle, magnet, electrical stimulation, or a laser beam, a shiatsu practitioner applies deep pressure, a practitioner of the Rolf technique stretches a layer of fascia, a sound therapist vibrates the tissue, a medical doctor uses a pulsating electromagnetic field, etc. The common denominator in all of these approaches is a living matrix that is exquisitely designed to absorb the information encoded in different kinds of vibratory energy and convert it into signals that are readily transmitted through the tensegrous semiconducting living matrix continuum.

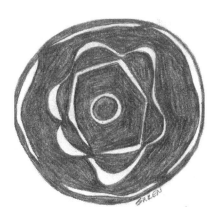

Artist's rendering of vibrational patterns created by spoken vowels (from Cymatics, *by Hans Jenny; see photo on page 51).*

Harold Saxton Burr was a pioneer in the study of energy fields in living systems. After earning his Ph.D. from Yale University in 1916, he remained there as a professor of anatomy for more than 40 years. His initial research centered on the nervous system, but after he found that he could measure and map the electric fields around living things with a standard voltmeter, he devoted his life to developing electrometric techniques that could be used in medical diagnosis and treatment. He demonstrated that a voltmeter could map the "electro-dynamic" field around every living thing, from mice to man, from seeds to trees. He called his discovery the fields of life, or L-fields. He believed that mapping distortions in a person's L-field can be useful in diagnosing pathological illnesses such as cancer, even before symptoms begin to develop.

In one study, Dr. Burr found a consistent, steady increase in the measured voltage in mice with developing cancer, whereas the control group showed no significant changes. Another study, at Bellevue Hospital in New York, detected a shift in voltage gradient, suggesting a malignancy, in 102 women who were being examined for ovarian cancer. Subsequent surgery confirmed 95 cases of malignancy.

Burr, working with psychiatrists, demonstrated that electrometric techniques are useful for distinguishing between normal and abnormal mental functions. He also showed that voltage recordings can indicate when ovulation is about to occur in women. Finally, he was able to measure voltage changes during the healing of wounds and showed that the changes could be correlated with the phases of healing.

Burr offered this explanation of L-fields: "Our bodies 'keep in shape' through ceaseless metabolism and changes of material. The mystery has been solved: the electro-dynamic field of the body serves as a matrix or mold which preserves the 'shape' or arrangement of any material poured into it, however often the material may be changed."

Life fields "regulate and control the creature whatever it may be and its aims are wholeness, organization and continuity," wrote Burr. "There is an organizational quality to these fields and they actually give rise to our physical bodies. If there is a mistake in this blueprint, a physical disease results. If you correct the blueprint you can correct physical disease."

In the 1940s, Reinhold Voll, a German physician, developed a device to measure the electrical parameters of acupuncture points. The Voll machine has been widely used to test responses to homeopathic remedies. Voll believed that tissue necrosis and organ degeneration decrease conductance along acupuncture paths, while inflammation increases conductance. Two British clinicians in the 1970s found that electrical conductance at the liver acupuncture point on the knees was 18 times greater in patients with inflamed livers than in subjects with no liver dysfunction. Another clinical study showed that electrical conduction at lung acupuncture points was 30 percent lower in patients with lung cancer than in healthy persons. Recently, computerized EDI (electro-dermal information) devices have been developed that are being used to identify homeopathic and vibrational remedies that correct imbalances that cause disease.

Homeopathy is regarded by many holistic healers as a form of vibrational medicine. In spite of the scorn heaped on homeopathy by most conventional medical practitioners in the U.S., its popular use continues to grow, and many stores now conveniently carry over-the-counter homeopathic remedies. Why so many people find that homeopathic remedies really work remains a mystery to the medical profession. Although many hospitals in the United States practiced homeopathic medicine in the late 1800s, "allopathic" physicians, who believed that drugs and surgery were the only legitimate forms of treatment, formed the American Medical Association (AMA) primarily to prevent the use of homeopathic medicine. Bylaws of the AMA prohibited fraternization with homeopathic practitioners or use of homeopathic remedies.

Samuel Hahnemann, a German physician, is credited with developing in the mid-1800s the healing principle that treating like with like can cure illnesses. This theory is similar in principle to vaccinations, which today are used worldwide. Homeopathic remedies usually are made from a plant or other substance in nature that produces in humans the symptoms of a particular illness. For instance, for colds and runny noses, a homeopathic remedy is made from onions.

In homeopathy, a potentially harmful substance is transformed into a medicine for healing by progressive dilution, until what remains is just the essence of the original substance. That essence contains the "memory" or energetic vibrations of the original substance. This idea is contrary to Western logic and medicine, since Western physicians believe that the larger the dosage, the stronger the effects. The idea that "less is more" is difficult for many people to grasp, despite the growing number of clinical studies that show that homeopathic remedies really work.

Often in homeopathy, the greater the dilution, the more potent the effect. A 100 x (one hundredfold) dilution is considered to be more potent than a 10 x dilution. How is it possible for a highly diluted remedy that contains only a few molecules of the original healing substance to be effective?

Physicists may eventually provide an answer. Molecules vibrate: they wiggle and jiggle. These vibrations are passed on to the surrounding molecules, transferring what physicists call "information." In addition, when a molecule absorbs an electromagnetic wave, it vibrates even more, sometimes so much that it emits another electromagnetic wave. This means that molecules may interact like a radio transmitter and receiver. Electromagnetic waves emitted by one molecule can be picked up by molecules "tuned in" to that frequency. If our radio telescopes are capable of detecting very weak electromagnetic waves from molecules billions of light years away from Earth, it is not improbable that our bodies have the means to detect signals emitted by only a few molecules.

The signals may be carried by certain electrons within a molecule. Physicists are only now learning how to manipulate a property of the electron known as "spin," which indicates its quantum state – either "up" or "down." It has been demonstrated that the spin of an electron can be transported without any loss of energy at room temperature. That may mean that "information" can be transferred by the electron from one molecule to another without energy loss. This emerging field of study is called spintronics. Scientists at

Stanford University are developing a sensitive electronic spin detector and hope to develop electronic devices in which spin current will flow without any energy loss.

Another answer is that homeopathic remedies do not work through the same physiological pathways that are activated by conventional drugs. Rather, homeopathy works by activating the resonant frequency of the patient. Jacques Benveniste, a homeopathic researcher in France, has provided exciting and dramatic evidence of electromagnetic resonance in dynamic living systems. He played recordings of the vibrational signals (in the human voice range) of typical messenger molecules in the human body and found that the messenger's normal receptors responded as if that molecule was actually present.

Even DNA may act as a resonant antenna. Rollin McCraty and Glen Rein of the HeartMath Institute in California (HeartMath.org) reported that DNA throughout the body receives and transmits information encoded within the heart's electrical rhythm. Information also appears to be contained within the oscillations of DNA. McCraty and his colleagues have examined the effects of rhythmic coherence on the molecular level in a living matrix and concluded that something like a piezoelectric effect may be present. The piezoelectric effect is reversible – pressure can be used to generate electricity, or electricity can be used to generate pressure.

Among other researchers, physicist Dan Winter has shown that there is a standing wave resonance of the heart and that physiological measurements are possible showing cardiac coherence (harmonically ordered – smooth sine waves). Winter has also created a beautiful array of computer graphics displaying the association of musical wave forms with emotions.

Our bodies are filled with oscillating fields – heartbeats, breath, brainwaves, the cerebrospinal fluid, vertebral acoustics. Our bodies also generate electromagnetic fields that communicate in direct currents, as demonstrated by Dr. Robert Becker and others. Becker noted that the body's direct-current system has a daily rhythm that seems to be tied to changes in the Earth's magnetic field.

Becker went on to show that applying external direct-current electricity accelerates the healing process in broken bones and tissues. He demonstrated that complete anesthesia can be induced by applying a magnetic field strong enough to change the activity of glial nerve cells. Becker's work laid the groundwork for a new field called neurotechnology, which uses electrical and magnetic impulses to directly stimulate specific sets of nerves to reduce chronic pain, to prevent epileptic seizures or Parkinson tremor, and to restore hearing. Other researchers have shown that applied electromagnetic fields can induce sleep, and a number of electrosleep devices are being marketed.

In 1952, the German physicist W.O. Schumann mathematically calculated that the cavity between the Earth's surface and the ionosphere, about 25 miles up, should have standing electromagnetic waves at certain frequencies. This is the same cavity that Nikola Tesla attempted to harness in the early 1900s. He tried to transmit electrical power through the air by activating the resonance of the cavity.

In 1954, the first electromagnetic standing wave in this cavity was detected and measured. Subsequently, additional standing-wave frequencies were detected. The strongest is at 7.8 Hz, with others at 14, 20, 26, 33, 39, and 45 Hz, the latter being the weakest. It is important to understand that these values are averages of readings from around the planet, and that the values vary daily by about 0.5 Hz. The standing waves become stronger when there is intense lightning activity. (Interestingly, a lightning strike generates an electromagnetic pulse that travels around the world about 7.4 times in one second.) The standing waves are also thought to be affected by sunspot activity, which peaks every 11 years.

These electromagnetic waves are now called Schumann resonances. The strongest standing wave, at 7.8 Hz, is thought to provide a timing signal to cells, which they use to maintain homeostasis, or optimal health. Indeed, several research studies have shown that all living cells resonate at the 7.8-Hz frequency. This Schumann resonance is also believed to have a direct effect on brain activity. In healthy humans, brainwaves at the 7.8-Hz frequency are associated with creative daydreaming or relaxed wakeful awareness. To many vibrational healers, the Schumann 7.8-Hz resonance acts like a tuning fork for human health.

Although we are bathed in the Earth's natural electromagnetic pulsations, we are also bombarded by stronger man-made electromagnetic waves. We are surrounded by electric wires that emit 50- or 60-Hz waves. Indoors and outdoors, we are immersed in high-frequency radio waves. Many believe this constant electromagnetic noise upsets the normal functioning of cells and systems in the body. We may be especially vulnerable to these permeating fields when we are in close proximity to microwave ovens, computers, and cell phones. Radiation from these devices may disrupt the body's direct-current communication system. I believe these vibrations, even though we do not hear them, do have a detrimental effect on our overall health.

The beating heart creates a standing wave of 7 Hz in the skeleton and skull, according to studies by Itzak Bentov, who summarized his findings in a chapter titled "Micromotion of the Body as a Factor of the Development of the Nervous System" in the book *Kundalini, Evolution and Enlightenment*, edited by John White. Using a device called a ballistocardiograph, Bentov found that a feedback exists between the heart and aortic bifurcation that creates a standing wave. During deep meditation, the timing of the pressure pulses traveling down the aorta is altered until it is in phase with the reflected pressure pulses from the bifurcation, and a standing wave with a frequency of 7 Hz is achieved.

This oscillation is transmitted to the skeleton, spine, and skull. The standing wave causes the brain to vibrate, creating several standing waves, which stimulate the ventricles and the sensory cortex of the brain. Bentov's innovative experiments led him to conclude that meditation activates five oscillators – the heart and four others – and locks them into rhythm: "When an individual achieves a deep state of meditation, breathing becomes slow and shallow and the heart activity becomes synchronized so as to create a resonant vibrational link between the heart and the brain. The oscillating electrical circuit within the brain becomes established only after gray matter along the sensory cortex has become completely polarized in a circular stimulus loop." This in turn produces a pulsating magnetic field around the head.

Bentov has clearly demonstrated that the nervous system can be entrained by the beating of the heart, and that resonant vibrational links exist throughout our bodies. Dan Winter came to a similar conclusion.

The true nature of the heart was revealed to me when I took a dissection anatomy class. I had separated some individual heart cells and saw that each cell beat independently of the others. But when I placed the heart cells closer together, they began beating as one. Their ability to synchronize and beat as one demonstrated to me the power of sympathetic vibrations.

To summarize, we have seen that the human body resonates to vibrations in ways that can promote healing. Some vibrations affect the body as a whole, while others affect only specific parts of the body. Vibrations are capable of altering individual cells and even molecules such as DNA. Furthermore, the body seems to be able to convert mechanical vibrations into wave-like electrical impulses, or convert electromagnetic waves into mechanical vibrations (the piezoelectric effect). Communication within the direct-current system discovered by Becker appears to be faster than that in the nervous system. All these research findings are puzzling to allopathic medical practitioners, who remain firm in their faith in drugs and surgery. Slowly, over the past several decades, a new and radical theory describing how the body and brain function has emerged. This new theory is based on the principle of holography and the idea that the brain and the body use a holographic process to recognize and to store information.

Holograms are unusual in that every part of the hologram contains the same information as the whole. In other words, you can cut the hologram into many pieces and each piece contains all the images that are contained in the hologram, but the smaller pieces will have less detail or definition.

Holography is a method of photography using a laser to provide coherent light – that is, light in which all of the waves are in order or synchronized. The beam of coherent light from a laser is split and part of the beam goes directly to the film. The second part of the beam is directed to the object to be holographed, and the reflected light is directed to the film through lenses. This scattered light is no longer coherent and interferes with the coherent beam that had been directed to the film. The resulting interference pattern is captured by the film, which contains all the information needed to reconstruct the image of the object. The astounding nature of the holograph is that the reconstructed image appears to be solid and three-dimensional.

Anything that behaves as a wave can be used to create an interference pattern. For example, when ripples on a pond cross other ripples moving in different directions, they create visible interference patterns. Both sound and electromagnetic waves, including light, can be used to create these patterns.

Carl Pribram, a neuroscientist at Stanford University in the 1960s, began thinking that memory may be stored in the brain in a holographic manner using wave fronts created by the firing of neurons. These wave fronts ripple through the brain, crossing each other and forming many interference patterns. It is these patterns that form the basis of memory, according to Pribram.

Before Pribram developed his holographic model, brain researchers generally believed that memory was stored in specific locales in the brain. Over the decades, however, many researchers, including Pribram, failed to find supporting evidence for the localization of memory. The renowned neuropsychologist Karl Lashley attempted to find the areas in brains of rats that contained memories related to learning to run a maze to get to food. To Lashley's surprise, no matter what portion of the brain he removed, some memory still remained. Even with massive parts of the brain removed, the rats continued to remember, although their motor skills were grossly impaired and they struggled awkwardly through the maze.

Pribram, who worked with Karl Lashley for a time, was puzzled by the evidence against localization of memory. Pribram reviewed medical cases involving patients who had had portions of the brain removed and found that there were no cases of selective memory loss. The patients' memories generally became hazy, but their memories were not lost completely. Even removal of a large portion of the temporal lobe did not create gaps in a person's memory. This further puzzled Pribram because Wilder Penfield, a neurosurgeon in Canada, appeared to have discovered in the 1920s that specific locations in the brain had specific memories. While performing open-brain surgery on epileptics, Penfield was able to evoke a specific memory in a patient by touching a certain spot on the temporal lobe. Thus stimulated, the patient seemed to relive an experience, much like movie flashback. When Pribram tried to duplicate Penfield's findings, this time in normal, non-epileptic patients, he was unable to evoke any specific memories.

To Pribram it now seemed that memories were not localized but were somehow distributed throughout the brain. When he became aware of holography (after reading an article in *Scientific American*), Pribram realized how distributed memory might work.

In his search through the scientific literature, Pribram came across the work of a Russian scientist, Nikolai Bernstein, who had discovered that physical movements are encoded in our brains as wave forms. Bernstein painted white dots on the black leotards of dancers and took movies of them in motion. In the films, the white dots appeared against a black background, so he could see how the movements flowed. To quantify his findings, he used Fourier analysis, a mathematical technique, to analyze the waveforms. According to the Fourier principle, every shape, no matter how complex, can be assembled or woven from a sum of pure sine waves.

Much to his surprise, Bernstein found that the Fourier analysis revealed wave forms with patterns that allowed him to predict the next movement within a fraction of an inch. Pribram recognized that Bernstein may have discovered how movement is stored in the brain. If the brain stores movement as wave forms, breaking them down into frequency components could help explain how we learn physical tasks. As Pribram put it, "The brain can instantly resonate to and thus recognize wave forms. Once recognized, the inverse transform allows them to be implemented into behavior."

The holographic theory applies not only to human learning, but also to memory and learning in animals, as well as memory in bacteria and lower animals that do not have a brain. Some recent studies of oscillation in cellular processes indicate that holographic information may be processed at the cellular and molecular levels.

The crossover design of the human visual and auditory systems suggests that something like holographic processing is occurring. The left visual field in each of the eyes is connected to the right side of the brain, while the right visual field goes to the left side of the brain. In the auditory system, some of the nerves in the ear are connected to the same side of the brain, and the remainder go to the opposite side. This is similar to the split-beam approach in holographic photography. In the case of the visual and auditory systems, the nerve impulses from one set of nerves act as reference beam to the impulses from the other side, resulting in a holographic interference pattern.

George J. Goodheart Jr., the chiropractor who originated the concept of applied kinesiology, proposes that the brain keeps a complete holographic image of every aspect of the body, and that if information from a local area does not match the holographic image, the brain takes notice. For instance, when the messages from a foot create a holographic pattern that does not match the one held by the brain, the cause is likely to be some kind of dysfunction. Goodheart has described how his holographic model can be useful in treating patients.

The holographic model also may provide an explanation for consciousness, for how we are able to be aware of ourselves. The holographic model makes it unnecessary to search for the seat of consciousness, or the location of a memory. I believe that consciousness is not just the result of neurons in firing in our brain, but rather an awareness that it resides in every cell and is manifested within all the systems of our bodies. This becomes more apparent when we view the body as a dynamic, energetic, interactive system.

James L. Oschman, in his book *Energy Medicine*, observes that when we take into account

> ... the biomagnetic fields of the organs and peripheral neurons, semiconduction through the cellular and sub-cellular structures associated with them, and the electromagnetic signatures of all the vibrating molecules within the cells and tissues, and we begin to see a dynamic picture of the energetic body as a whole. What we refer to as 'mind' and 'consciousness' may encompass the totality of communications and regulations in the body, the electromagnetic signatures of countless molecules and atoms, and the energy fields they entail. ... Emerging concepts of consciousness have profound therapeutic implications.

Standing waves are found throughout nature and within our bodies. The heart, the brain, and the spine are oscillating systems based on simple, harmonic standing waves. When the vibratory fields in the heart, brain, and nervous system are in phase, augmenting each other harmoniously using the heart and the vertebrae as conductors, coherent messages can then be produced, culminating in consciousness.

CHAPTER 11

FUTURE DIRECTIONS

WHETHER YOU ARE A CHIROPRACTOR, osteopathic physician, physical therapist, holistic doctor, acupuncturist, massage therapist, or vibrational healer, you can utilize bone toning today in your practice. Treatments can be done with either tuning forks or a frequency generator. For treating the vertebrae of the spine, the resonant frequencies for each vertebra can be found in Chapter 6. Other vibrational healers have developed methods for treating other parts of the body, and many are willing to supply the proper tuning forks and tools.

Additional research is needed to refine and extend the use of spinal bone toning. With the aid of a tunable, hand-held frequency generator, it will be possible to accumulate vertebra frequency data from a larger population. Investigations of patients with spinal injuries may lead to new diagnostic procedures with tunable vibrators.

It may be possible that an instrument can be developed to complement or replace muscle testing. For instance, the PulStar FRAS and the Nervo-scope have the potential to be adapted to measure muscle and nerve response.

Physicians, scientists, and researchers are just beginning to glimpse the healing powers of sound and are only scratching the surface with regard to its potential use. My hope for the future is that hospitals and clinics will employ healing forms of music, sound, and light in their treatment rooms and will begin to use other forms of vibrational medicine to help their patients bring the body/mind/spirit back to balance.

Hospitals surely have their place. If I were severely injured in a car accident, I certainly would want to be taken to a hospital emergency room. But if I am being treated by a doctor for an illness or dysfunction, I would prefer a doctor who wholeheartedly supports a holistic approach to health care. I would like to see more support in the medical community for non-invasive treatments, and more grants for research in the area of vibrational and energy medicine.

Time-reversed acoustics using ultrasonic pulses has proven to be effective in locating and breaking up kidney stones (see Chapter 9). A modified form of time-reversed acoustics may make it possible to treat specific vertebrae and nerves in a variety of conditions, including osteoporosis and degenerative joint disease. In such cases, sonic pulses that echo from a vertebra and its surrounding tissue can be time-reversed and sent back. The vertebra and tissue may resonate with time-reversed sound waves and perhaps regain normal function to some extent. It is possible that research with time-reversed vibrations may lead to new vibrational therapies.

Ancient mythology refers to sound as the primordial substance from which our universe originated. Recent photographs by satellites of the far reaches of the universe have revealed that sound indeed was present in the primordial plasma, and sound created the temperature differences that led to the formation of matter. Both the ancient Sanskrit Vedas and the Bible refer to sound as the heart of all existence.

Chladni and Jenny demonstrated that for every sound, there is a corresponding shape or pattern that can be seen as the effect of the vibration on a powder or liquid. Research showed that when Tibetan monks chanted the sound of OM, a resonator plate formed a pattern known as Sri Yantra, which Hindus believe is the creation pattern of the universe. Stan Tenen of the Meru Foundation analyzed recorded wave patterns formed by the spoken sounds of the Hebrew alphabet and found a correlation between the shapes of the wave patterns and the shapes of the letters in the alphabet.

Sound is being used to treat geopathic stresses such as pollution and other environmental dysfunctions. Some researchers have broadcast certain sound frequencies to counteract air pollution. In the Cape Flats area of South Africa, delivery of sonic vibrations with a series of harmonizers reportedly decreased pollution by 50 percent within hours! (For more information, contact Christian Hummel through www.earthtransitions.com.)

Rainforests appear to maintain the acoustic balance in their territory. According to the bioacoustic habitat theory, if a species in a particular area dies off, the forest quickly replaces the spectrum of its sounds. An underlying premise is that the sounds of insects and animals are crucial to the survival of their ecosystem. One study found that bird songs stimulate plants to bloom and to grow more rapidly. In Australia, a researcher found that the symphony of sounds made by frogs, crickets, and other insects appeared to induce rainfall in the area. Other Australian researchers discovered that the pattern of coral reefs is shaped at least in part by the sounds of dolphins.

Perhaps one day we shall discover the sacred sounds or chants that will change the course of human events so that peace shall prevail.

OM

SHALOM

Chapter 12

THE DANCE OF LIFE

A Jack of all trades
A master of none,
My mother says

Who am I to deny a part of myself
I am a master of adaptability
I can be anything
Because
I am part of everything

I'm just a lover of life
With a passion to live
As I close these tired eyes to rest
I feel a fullness
A richness
I have been given another opportunity
Another lesson
Another gift

Upon awakening to the morning sun
And a bird's song, I am empty
Ready to embrace another day

Come join me my friends, in the celebration
Of this wondrous, rhythmic, graceful dance
Called …
Life

– June Leslie Wieder

(The highest form of prayer is gratitude.
Thank you, God.)

SUGGESTED READINGS AND OTHER SOURCES

(By no means is a comprehensive list)

Ackerman, Diane	*History of the Senses*
	The Moon by Whale Light
Beaulieu, John	*Music and Sound in the Healing Arts*
Becker, Robert and Gary Selden	*The Body Electric*
Benade, Arthur H.	*Fundamentals of Musical Acoustics*
	Horns, Strings, and Harmony
Bentov, Itshak	*Stalking the Wild Pendulum: On the Mechanics of Consciousness*
Berendt, Joachim-Ernst	*Nada Brahma: The World Is Sound*
Campbell, Don	*The Mozart Effect*
	Music: Physician for Times to Come
Carey, Donna and Marjorie de Muynck	*There's No Place Like Ohm*
Diamond, John	*Your Body Doesn't Lie*
Gerber, Richard	*Vibrational Medicine*
Goldman, Jonathan	*Healing Sound*
	Shifting Frequencies
Greene, Brian	*The Elegant Universe*

Hart, Mickey	*Drumming on the Edge of Magic*
Hawkins, David	*Power vs. Force*
Helmholtz, Hermann	*On the Sensations of Tone*
Jenny, Hans	*Cymatics: A Study of Wave Phenomena and Vibrations*
Jourdain, Robert	*Music, the Brain, and Ecstasy*
Juhan, Deane	*Job's Body: A Handbook for Bodywork*
Kahn, Hazrat Inayat	*The Music of Life*
Keyes, Laurel Elizabeth	*Toning, The Creative Power of the Voice*
Leeds, Joshua	*The Power of Sound* *Sonic Practitioners*
Leonard, George	*The Silent Pulse*
Linklater, Kristin	*Freeing the Natural Voice*
Liskin, Jack	*Moving Medicine*
Melchizedek, Drunvalo	*The Ancient Secret of the Flower of Life, Vols. 1 and 2*
Oschman, James L.	*Energy Medicine: The Scientific Basis*
Scaravelli, Vanda	*Awakening the Spine*
Schwenk, Theodor	*Sensitive Chaos: The Creation of Flowing Forms In Water and Air*
Tomatis, Alfred	*The Conscious Ear*
Trager, Milton	*Trager Mentastics*

Videos

Of Sound, Mind & Body: Music and Vibrational Healing

Cymatics – The Healing Nature of Sound

Cymatic Soundscapes

Available from Jeff Volk
MACROmedia
219 Grant Road
Newmarket, New Hampshire 03857
www.cymaticsource.com

Healing Sounds: Principles of Sound Healing

Available from Jonathan Goldman
www.healingsounds.com

RECOMMENDED WEBSITES

Acutonics (www.acutonics.com)

Cymatics (www.cymatics.org.uk, www.cymaticsource.com)

The Healing Music Organization (www.healingmusic.org)

Holographic Repatterning (www.holographic.org)

Trager (www.trager.com, www.trager-us.org)

Dr. John Beaulieu (www.biosonics.com)

Jonathan Goldman (www.healingsounds.com)

Joshua Leeds (www.appliedmusic.com, www.sound-remedies.com)

Fabian Maman (www.tama-do.com)

Dr. Jeffrey Thompson — Center for Neuroacoustic Research (www.neuroacoustic.com)

Dr. June Leslie Wieder (www.drwieder.com, www.bone-toning.com)

~ NOTES ~

~ NOTES ~

~ NOTES ~

Made in the USA
San Bernardino, CA
19 May 2018